CW01481515

# Make Her Scream: La Come Harder, and Be ⊓ιc ⊔cσι She's Ever Had

## By Amber Cole, Sex Coach

# Table of Contents

# 1. Inside the female mind.

There are countless differences between men and women.

As much as we'd all like to believe in the ideal of equality, there are biological limits to it.

This isn't just limited to how we look, our physical capabilities, and how much muscle we can build. It also impacts our **psychology** in many areas of our lives.

One such area is, of course, **sex**.

There are day-and-night differences between the male mind and the female mind as far as love and sex are concerned. Guys who want to understand women sexually have to wrap their minds around this.

If you want to be a better lover or attend to the physical needs of your partner more effectively, you have to understand these differences. Understand the contents of this chapter and let it reflect in how you treat her.

The biology of love and sex.

The psychological impact as far as sex is concerned is greatly influenced by evolution.

Males produce sperm. Sperm is produced by the millions every single day.

Females produce eggs. Eggs, on the other hand, take a lot of energy to produce and females only produce a limited quantity of them and depending on how her reproductive system is functioning; they only produce one egg per month.

The implication is very straightforward.

Males need as many as sexual partners as possible because they have the sperm to service all those partners. The goal of the male is to impregnate as many women as possible. I'm talking about the evolutionary impact on the biology of the male human mind.

This impacts male behavior. The more sex partners, the better because that's how they have been taught biologically. The female, on the other hand, spends all this energy producing one egg. She is looking for the top male and for quality males who would produce the best sperm to fertilize this one egg.

It's like an **investment game**.

If you poured all of your life savings into one asset, you're going to be very, very careful where to invest that asset, how to grow that asset, and who to trust with that asset.

On the other hand, if you produce tons of money every single day, you're more liberal with your money. You're more willing to spend it on anything that comes to mind. Males want to impregnate as many different women as possible. They don't really care who it is, as long as they get their seed out there.

As you can already tell, there is going to be a clash between the female mind and the male mind as far as sexual reproduction is concerned. **This is where love comes in**.

**Love is a filtering mechanism**.

The whole concept of love is that it binds people together in an emotional manner so that they protect each other. Love as a concept greatly favors females because if we are going to follow the male psychological model, there would be no need for love because the whole point of sex would be to have sex with as many partners as possible.

This flies completely in the face of the concept of love. Love is all about two people, in the same place, providing support for each other.

The females need this because of their one egg. The egg

develops into a fetus which develops into a child. The child takes a long time to physically mature. All that time, that child would need food, shelter, and protection.

This is where the male needs to be in the picture.

How do you keep them in the picture? The concept of love and loyalty. If you were just going to follow the psychological implications of the biological make-up of men, this wouldn't make any sense because it would be in his advantage to just spread his seed out there.

But love exists, and love is our countervailing model against raw sex drive.

The wake of society determines the proper ways to express desire and opening yourself up sexually, and is influenced by this interplay between the male sex drive and the female focus on love.

Don't get me wrong, women want sex.

Sex is a key part of their psychology. However, it is in its proper context. It has to move within the orbit of the biological and psychological truths I just explained earlier.

On the one hand, they can't just go with their sex drive because there is this built in biological impulse to be very selective regarding their sexual partner. On the other hand, they are also working with the societal and cultural factors that reinforce that selectivity. More traditional cultures say they shouldn't have sex until they get married.

Some cultures even restrict that choice even further. The third factor that they are dealing with is the fact that they are swarmed by guys who just want to have sex.

So, this is the female mindset and how they navigate that is crucial to their development of a healthy attitude towards sex. You, on the other hand, looking at them from the outside, must understand how this process works and ultimately, make it work to your favor.

## 2. What females value in sex differs from what men value.

One of the most common rookie mistakes that guys make when it comes to sexual relationships is that they assume women like what they like and what women value in sex is identical to what they want.

Bad move.

If you are approaching women this way, you are doomed to fail. You have to understand that even though women want sex and in many cases, and often with the same intensity as men, there are limits as to how they express that desire.

Moreover, they have to work with cultural barriers, societal barriers, physical barriers, so on and so forth. So even if it's true that the desire is there, the expression of that desire and what is acceptable and unacceptable is very different between men and women.

Guys who ignore this fact are basically playing the sex game to lose. If you want to be more successful in not just attracting women sexually but also pleasing them sexually, you have to understand how females value sex.

<u>The focus on trust and security.</u>

As I mentioned earlier, there is no difference in sexual desire between men and women.

The problem is the layers on top of that desire and how sexual attraction is expressed in what is deemed acceptable or unacceptable. Moreover, a very important difference is in motivation.

Women value sex because they feel secure when they're with a man. This requires a lot of trust. Again, there's a huge amount of biological evolution involved in this. As I've mentioned in the previous chapter, women only produce one egg. That egg can lead to an offspring, and this is why the woman needs to protect that egg. That's her only investment.

Guys, on the other hand, produce millions upon millions of sperm every single day. Guys really don't have that much of a vested interest in protecting their sperm because they know on an unconscious biological level that they can produce another batch of millions the next day and the day after that.

Women, however, have only one bite at the apple once

every month. Security, protection, reassurance, and related values are very important to women as far as sex is concerned. This is then reflected in the need for trust. Before you get women into bed, they're looking to trusting you first.

Guys focus on availability. As long as the female is available, it's good to go. Of course, every guy is different. Different guys have different standards and different thresholds, but the underlying reality is the same. With women, it starts with trust, which is a reflection of a deep and profound need for security.

Women value comfort.

If you are going to invest all your time and energy into one asset, you need somebody to protect you and give you the level of comfort you need to make sure that asset grows. That asset, as far as women are concerned, is our children.

Attitudes forged over hundreds of thousand of years of evolution are very hard to shake. There is a profound need on the part of women to focus on comfort as far as sex is concerned. The guy must be able to make them comfortable. Evolutionary speaking, a guy must have the physical means to provide for a family and make sure that their needs are met.

Women don't like to be in charge.

A lot of feminists would have a problem with this, but if we are just going to look the biological impact on modern psychology, we have to conclude that women don't like to be in charge. They are looking for alpha males.

We had to look back tens of thousands or hundreds of thousands of years ago and if the scientists are correct, human beings follow the same mating patterns as other mammals. What mating pattern is that? Winner takes all. When you look at most mammals, it's the alpha male – the aggressive dominant male – who gets the only chance and right to have sex with all the females in the group.

When you look at prides and prides of lions, that's how it works.

This impacted women's psychology on a subconscious level and it persists today. It persists in one very simple form: Women don't like to be in charge sexually. They are always looking for signs of guys who are in charge, and they are attracted to that guy.

The role of romance in sex for women.

Romance, on its face, seems to have overturned a lot of these harsh biological realities. The whole focus on love seems to contradict the very basic male drive to spread sperm as far and wide as possible but in reality, the same factors are still in play.

As you probably already know, hundreds of thousands of

years of biology are very hard to reverse. In fact, modern human economy and modern human technology can really just be traced to maybe a few hundred years. We still have a long way to go if we want to reverse the biological cement that our destinies are imprinted in.

Regardless, the role of romance and sex for women focuses on the need for trust, security, comfort, and not being in charge.

The role of the guy is to be emotionally intimate during sex. Your job is to not just follow your biological wiring and just do a quick in and out and get out of there. There has to be an emotional intimacy there and an emotional dance.

In a way, this is kind of how human beings mirror the mating patterns of birds. Have you ever watched the Nature channel or Animal Planet and watched birds mate? They go through elaborate dances. They send all sorts of complicated signals to each other to signify receptivity. Once the male does the right dances, then the female allows him to mate with her.

The same applies to human beings but instead of physical dances, which can also take place on the dance floor, we're talking primarily about emotional dances which you have to go through. These are emotional hoops that you need to jump through to send the right signals so that she can be ready physically.

We're talking about looking into her eyes, holding her hands, whispering in her ear, touching her in the right places, caressing her, taking her to a secluded area and making her feel that she's the center of your world, making her feel comfortable, prized, and appreciated.

The list is very long, but it all leads to one place.

All these rituals have a central point. The central point is you need to express physical actions that build trust, security, comfort, and show to her, in no uncertain terms, that you are in charge. That's all there is to it. These signals get her ready for the physical act of sex. If you don't go through all these hoops, she won't be ready.

### 3. The art of seduction.

When most people hear the word "seduction," all sorts of images come to mind.

They think you have to be very slick with women, have some sort of magic pick up lines, and go through these steps to get women into bed.

While there's some truth to that, most people lose sight of a larger truth.

The larger truth is that if you want to persuade people to do what you want them to do, you are engaging in seduction. Defined this way, seduction is happening all the time everywhere. Whether you're trying to sell detergent, TV sets, sound systems, or trying to get people to click on your link on your Facebook and all points in between, you're engaged in the art of seduction.

Seduction is really all about sending off the right signals verbally, non-verbally, textually, digitally, or whatever it is to get people to do what you want them to do. That is seduction.

Many guys fail to get women into bed because they let the whole concept of seduction get the best of them. They are intimidated by the whole prospect of seducing women. They think that it takes too much for it or there is some sort of magic formula or arcane process that they need to master so they can get women to do their bidding.

There seems to be an almost Karate Kid Mister Miyagi type of mystique to the art of seduction.

Get all those ideas out of your mind.

If you know how to sell, guess what? You have 90% of sexual seduction nailed. If you know how to write an essay, you're doing even better. You got 95% of the art of seduction pinned down. The art of seduction really is all about persuasion. What makes sexual seduction different from the other types of persuasion, both written and unwritten, is that it involves a lot of non-verbal signals.

Most people really fail in seduction simply because of inconsistency.

If they put themselves in front of the mirror, and they are trying to convince their reflection to do something, they would realize that their facial expressions, their tone of voice, their body language, and their aura are off and do not match the content of their words. It's no surprise that they fail in persuading people.

If people noticed a distinct break in what you're doing compared to what you're saying, people won't take you seriously. At the very least, people are confused. What do people do when they're confused? They don't do anything and freeze up.

What this means then in terms of sexual seduction is being mindful and managing the overall signals you're sending to the person who is the target of your desires. Keep the following in mind so you can increase your ability to seduce women.

Make her feel beautiful and wanted.

I want you to read that subheading once again. The keyword is "feel." That's very important. It's not about what you feel, what you think, or what you want. It's all about what she feels. Many guys fail to do this because they focus primarily on what they want. Granted we're all self-absorbed and self-centered people; we're all selfish.

You need to fight against that and set that aside if you want to be successful in seducing women. You have to step out of yourself. You have to make another person the center of your world at least for the next few minutes. The key here is to focus on what she feels.

What kind of signals can you send out to make her feel

beautiful and wanted? What kind of facial expressions, tone of voice, and body language can you project and radiate out so she can feel appreciated and valued? That's a puzzle that you need to solve on an individual basis because everybody's physical signals are different.

Make sure that the physical signals that you are sending out are very easy to read and more importantly, not confusing. In many cases, all you need to do is stand in front of the mirror and stay stuff. The words that you say have a particular meaning but how you say it may lead to another meaning. There has to be a perfect consistency between what you say and how you say it.

Keep practicing. This is how you make her feel beautiful and wanted when the signals you're sending out are unmistakable.

Discover her love language.

There are five love languages.

They are: (1) being told sweet and pleasant things, (2) giving gifts, (3) physical contact and touch, (4) performing acts of service, and (5) quality conversation and time.

This is how people detect love, and this is how they show love.

If you want to seduce a woman, you need to discover very quickly what her love language is. Does she like to be touched, be told reassuring stuff, like small gifts, so on and so forth? The good news is that she'll probably do this for you. How? By showing her love language to you.

If you noticed that the woman you're interested in likes to give small gifts, guess what? That's her love language. You need to give her small gifts as well.

Learn her fantasies.

You need to get under her skin and really draw her out. Learn what her fantasies are. The good news is that all women have fantasies. Your job is to learn which ones they are. You should then revisit them and tell stories that involve those fantasies. Maybe you need to couch how you communicate with her based on how they appeal to her fantasies.

The reason why you need to learn her fantasies is because they reflect her ideals. They reflect how she views a perfect courtship. By changing the way you communicate to better fit this ideal, the better you look in her eyes.

The only potential issue here is that you must proceed slowly because she may fear judgment. You simply need to reassure her that you are extremely non-judgmental, and create a safe space for her vulnerability. Sharing one of your deeper fantasies and philias often makes her feel less judged, because if you can share with her, she will open up too.

<u>The end goal is to make her want you.</u>

The whole point of the art of seduction is to make her want you. That's right. You as an individual. You, specifically.

## 4. Teasing: stoking the flames in the buildup.

In the chapter on seduction, I have painted in broad strokes what you need to do to get a female to open her mind about having sex with you.

Now, we're going to get a little bit more specific. Seduction is a long and drawn-out process. It covers many areas in your relationship or future relationship with this woman. It impacts a lot of the communications and mental images that you would have about each other.

Foreplay, on the other hand, is more specific. It's all about one thing and one thing alone: the sex act.

A lot of guys really drop the ball when it comes to foreplay because they think that foreplay is just all about getting the oven ready so you can put in the stuff you need to bake. I'm sorry but if that is your definition of foreplay, you are probably going to be looked at as a very lousy lover.

Foreplay is physical, yes, but there are emotional layers on top of it. You have to remember that you are dealing with women. Women are emotional creatures.

With women, the physical component of foreplay has to be wrapped in the think layer of emotional seduction. The whole point of foreplay is to build up to penetration. It's very easy to lose sight of this.

It's like being led to a candy store, and you see a hallway of candy and at the end of the hallway; you see that nice, thick stack of Hershey's chocolate or Reese's peanut buttercups that you came into the store for in the first place. Your initial tendency, if you're a normal person, is to basically just rush through that aisle to stuff your face with the chocolate at the end of the aisle. You should resist that temptation.

Instead of just sticking it in and getting it over with, you have to understand that there are two people engaged in sex. It's not just you. This is really the biggest challenge as far as foreplay is concerned.

Most guys would rather rush through foreplay. They think that it's just a necessary price they have to pay, like paying a toll in a highway. But if you want to be invited back to the party, you need to master foreplay, and the key part here is your mindset. Your mindset is to learn how to enjoy giving of yourself and to enjoy putting the needs of another person before your own.

The good news is that it's very easy to get used to foreplay.

For this chapter, we're going to discuss foreplay in the context of teasing. As I've mentioned earlier, foreplay is physical, emotional and psychological. In this chapter, we're talking primarily about the emotional and psychological layers. You have to build her up to open her up.

<u>Texting and sexting.</u>

To psychologically get your partner ready for sex, you need to make her feel wanted. You have to get her excited about what you're going to be doing together. Text her caring, romantic, and sweet statements. This turns women on; guys somewhat less so.

You need to be in the same psychological space with your partner for everything else to line up and the sex to be meaningful to her.

For guys, sex is always meaningful because it leads to ejaculation. That's really the only benchmark for men as far as what good sex is. You ejaculate at the end. With women, it's harder and the key part of that is laying the psychological groundwork. Get her psychologically excited so she can get emotionally excited, which then triggers physical arousal.

Once she responds to your text that communicates intimacy, desire, and appreciation, the next step is to sext.

You send messages that involve sexual imagery. I'm not talking about being nasty and saying, "I want to donkey fuck you."

No. I'm talking about physically suggestive text, like "I miss nibbling on your ear" or "I miss the taste of your lips," that kind of text message.

The difference is physical intimacy.

Again, if you push the envelope too far and just say, "I just want to fuck or I just want to bend you over," you strip away the emotional intimacy, and you make it like a raw and primal exercise in sex. Some women dig this. Some women get wet thinking about this stuff, but most women will find it repulsive.

So you need again to understand how seduction works and take small steps towards the goal. You're going to get there. No need to rush down that aisle and stuff your face with those Hershey bars. You need to walk slowly through the candy aisle. I know it's very tempting, but you need to go through these hoops.

When you feel comfortable, jump into texting and exchanging dirty pictures with each other. You will likely have to start this process because women are notoriously self-conscious about their bodies. Once you jumpstart the process, it will prompt her to reciprocate. Shirtless pictures work well to start with, and then you can start moving to more explicit areas.

Word of advice: a good rule of thumb is to not include your face with your genitals! This is good practice in the age of the Internet, and protecting your identity and future in case things go south.

<u>Dirty talkin'.</u>

The whole point about sexting is it's all about escalating polite, nice text to nastier and nastier messages. The whole point here is to communicate to her that you want her and desire on a physical AND emotional level.

Most guys don't really have a problem with dirty talk. It's just a question of scaling it up properly so it doesn't come off as offensive.

But just in case you want some guidelines...

First, tell her what you want to do with her and be specific. For example, "I'm going to bend you over like a bad girl."

Second, tell her what you want her to do to you and be specific. For example, "I want you to get on your knees and ask me what I want."

Third, brush up on your dirty vocabulary and make sure that you can say filthy words without giggling or cracking a smile.

Finally, ask her questions that you know the answer will be "yes" to. For example, "You like when I pull your hair hard?"

To heck with guidelines, how about an entire huge section on dirty talk?

Even with the realizations that we've reached in the previous chapter, it can be tough to simply open your mouth and utter those things. Logic has nothing to do it with it, and self-consciousness and potential judgment everything.

We can have all the justification in the world to do something, but that's not what determines our actions in daily life... as many of us are far too familiar with.

Even if I give you the perfect phrases to whisper, they will be useless until you can actually work up to whispering or shouting them during orgasm.

Simply put, the first time you try anything new, you will feel that self-consciousness and adrenaline rush of uncertainty. It is unavoidable. But there are steps you can take to reduce those feelings and turn them into excitement and arousal.

Hell, you might even skip over a couple of the following steps because you've acclimated more quickly than you expected – and that's what I find with most people. The important thing here is that everyone moves along at their own pace of comfort, and no one can be expected to follow someone else's and move together exactly.

So if your partner is lagging, guess what... go back and help them!

### Step one – bring it up innocently

First, talk about dirty talk with your partner. Bring it up innocuously and gauge their reaction to it. Tell them that a friend told you about it, and you were intrigued, so that the burden can be blamed on someone else. Or say that you read an article about it, saw a television piece on it, etc. You can also watch something together that has elements of dirty talk so the topic comes up independently of you.

Bringing it up this way gives you an out and plausible deniability so you can avoid self-consciousness and judgment. Your partner most likely will not be judging you, but this is an approach that helps you justify talking about it.

I would estimate that 99% of the time, your partner will be intrigued and agreeable to trying whatever you suggest in the name of spicing up bedroom relations. If they aren't, they might simply be in the same shoes you are – afraid of judgment and self-conscious about their sexuality. If that's the case, you need to move along slowly and emphasize that you are interested in exploring it.

You might need to bring the topic up more than once for it to truly implant in your partner's head.

If they are truly reluctant to give it a shot, there's not much you can do except continue to keep communication lines open and extoll the virtues of dirty talk.

Do *not* push them into something they don't want to try.

### Step two – learn your vocabulary

Don't dive into using dirty talk during sex yet.

You need to focus on the two main components of dirty talk – *vocabulary, and action phrases.*

As you'll see, you will need to be comfortable and proficient with both of them. Get used to using various vocabulary words such as "cock," "pussy," "tight," "soaked," "fuck me" and so on. *Think* about how you can use them in your daily life to get over any prevailing stigma you might feel from them.

Roll them around your tongue and mouth them – you don't need to outright say or use them yet. You can do the same with action phrases such as "I'm going to," "spread yourself," "bend over," "pound me," and the like. Whisper them to yourself and become comfortable with them.

You are becoming a person who is a dirty talk expert, and that requires changing your mindset and expanding your comfort zones.

Make sure that you are also ridding yourself of your daily usage of lesser dirty talk words like "wiener," "dick," "vagina," and so on. Those are kiddy words. They have no place in dirty talk.

### Step three – writing and typing it

Third, test these phrases and vocabulary out via text or instant messaging. Actually writing these out will be adrenaline-inducing for the first few times, but you'll find that the initial hurdle... is really the only hurdle there is. The first time is the hardest, and each time you use anything you'll be exponentially more comfortable with it. Once you see that there is no negative reaction, that's going to be a powerful piece of positive reinforcement to keep pushing the envelope!

If you need an intermediate step between steps two and three, I suggest seeking out an online chatroom geared towards cybersex and dirty talk. For some, this skirts a moral grey area, but it's in the name of love! Try out your phrases anonymously and without fear of retribution and judgment! The goal is just to get used to actually using them on someone, and seeing the proper context and reactions that people will have. You might even pick up a few tips while you're there.

Once you've mastered using your phrases and vocabulary via the written word, you can try trotting them out in person in the next step.

### Step four – introduce outside of the bedroom

Fourth, now that you're comfortable with all the phrases and words and actually have used them to some degree, try using them in a joking manner with your partner *out loud… not during sex*. Take away the stigma and the embarrassment by saying everything with a wry smirk, and get used to saying the words and their reactions.

You'll get a chance for feedback, practice, and to discover what your partner particularly likes or does not like. Watch some amateur pornography for inspiration on how to use dirty talk naturally and organically. If you're still having trouble, try finding some audiobooks of erotica or erotic stories online – you can see exactly what kind of tone and inflection that you can use.

The goal in this step is to get used to saying the vocabulary and phrases with your partner orally to find out what they like and build comfort.

### Step five – transition to sex

Finally, transition into the bedroom. At this point, you should have no issues saying that you want to say because you've already taken away the mystique of the words in other contexts. You should also realize at this point that there will be no judgment on your partner's part. This is key.

It will be slightly nerve-wracking because it is a new

context, but you'll have these phrases at the tip of your tongue and instinctually realize when to use them for maximum arousal.

Start with moaning and groaning louder and more emphatically than normal.

Then continue by incorporating dirty talk phrases into your moaning and groaning. Practice makes perfect!

You may find that you have to do the majority of the leading and dirty talking when you first begin with your partner, so be prepared for it.

The wonderful part about dirty talk is that you have probably been playing a waiting game – that is, your partner didn't want to be the first person to bring it up, and is thankful that you did it. Discovering shared secret interests, especially those of the dirty nature, can be a huge aphrodisiac in itself.

The phrase "It's not what you say, but how you say it" has rarely mattered more than with dirty talk. I can feed you the phrases to use (and I will later), but there are a few guidelines that we have to cover in the delivery of your dirty talk. Of course, part of this is practice and realizing what works for you and your partner.

Delivery is key for dirty talk because of the overall mood and tone you are seeking to cultivate.

### Giggle attacks

First, we have to talk about giggling.

This is the first guideline for a reason. Everyone, me included, will occasionally suffer from giggle attacks from delivering dirty talk. There's not much I can say to prevent, but I can try to emphasize the mood-killing effect of it.

When you yourself giggle during the *delivery* of dirty talk, it potentially ruins the mood of the entire sexual experience.

Instead of having a transcendent set of orgasms, giggling imparts the mood of just fooling around and laughing... which is not how anyone would describe passion. The best orgasm you've ever had – I bet you weren't laughing before it. The steamiest, hottest sex you've had – I bet jokes weren't a component. We're aiming for raw, primal passion, and a case of the giggles simply breaks that path.

The next time you're on the verge of giggling during your delivery, just bite your tongue until the moment passes.

And giggling from *receiving* dirty talk from your partner? Now that's a crushing blow in two ways: to their confidence in their dirty talk skills, and to the mood that they are trying to cultivate. Avoid that at all costs. In the same vein, never criticize their dirty talk or make them feel bad about it until after the session.

## *Eye contact*

Eye contact is a powerful tool in all walks of life, so it's only natural that it should be paired with expert dirty talk. Whenever possible, pair dirty talk with eye contact, regardless of whether you are receiving or delivering it.

If you are in a situation (or position) in which you aren't facing each other at the moment but feel the need to deliver some dirty talk, take a moment's pause from whatever you doing, seek eye contact (or outright grab their face), and say it. It's a power move that will enhance the words coming out of your mouth, and make your partner want you that much more... and return to the task at hand with renewed vigor and lust.

Whispering dirty talk into someone's ear from behind or from the front is one of the only acceptable times where eye contact would not necessarily enhance the phrases.

If you find that you have trouble with eye contact in general walks of life, I have a practice tip for you. Put on a pair of sunglasses, and take a stroll around your block. Make eye contact with people that you walk across with impunity, because they can't see your eyes. It's like viewing them through a one-way mirror! Notice how many people make only a spit-second of eye contact, or avoid it altogether.

This exercise is to realize that eye contact is easier than you think, and that other people also have trouble with it.

### Fake it 'til you make it

As with many things in life, people will become comfortable with dirty talk only when they can sense that you are also comfortable with it. For example, if someone is extremely self-deprecating and depressed, that makes the people around him uncomfortable because they simply don't know how to react.

Dirty talk embodies that feeling of mutual comfort. If your partner can sense that you are uncomfortable with the things you are saying, it will diminish the experience and decrease their comfort and enjoyment levels intensely.

It's unavoidable for us to 100% comfortable and confident in our dirty talk skills the first few times around, so my advice here is simply to fake that comfort and confidence until it becomes real. Whisper or demand things in a strong and clear tone of voice, and don't let on that you are way out of your comfort zone... because then you will take them out of theirs.

Don't utter something then ask if that was okay or embarrassing.

Own it.

Whisper, state, demand, and scream confidently!

### Background music fills the gaps

Even though this is obviously a book on the virtues of dirty talk, I should make it clear that I'm not suggesting that your sexual encounters be like a Gilmore Girls episode – non-stop chatter and banter.

Playing music in the background will help reduce the need to fill the space with dirty chatter. It's also a good intermediate step for beginners, as having the background noise will make novices less self-conscious about what they're saying.

At first, turn the music on loudly so your partner will barely hear your words, but you get acclimated to using them during actual sex. Gradually turn the music volume down, and you've just gradually conditioned yourself to be less self-conscious with dirty talk.

On another note, playing background music during sex is great for setting the mood and tone of the sex itself... which will influence the type of dirty talk that you whip out.

Boyz 2 men? Get ready for a steamy session with lots of slow kissing and grinding.

Rammstein? Well...

### Warm up then ramp up

Just like most sexual experiences, dirty talk should start more slow and tame... and then ramp up to dirty and downright filthy when the intensity of the sex picks up.

During any sexual encounter, there are necessary phases of arousal that we all go through. This is both a mental and physical process that culminates in an erection or adequate lubrication. Sometimes we go through it quickly and even skip a phase or two, but more often than not, we proceed through each stage methodically.

It's a time-tested process that heightens arousal and sets an individual's mood. If you are disturbed from that process that you are used to, you risk being taken out of the mood entirely.

You wouldn't try shoving your cock into her while she's barely wet, would you? You can't shove your mindcock into her brainpussy when it's barely lubed up either.

Skew to using more tender and gentle dirty talk at first, and save your filthy mouth for later when your partner will be able to appreciate it the most. This segues into my next point nicely.

### Calibrate to your partner

As I discussed before, everyone has their set pattern and phases of arousal that they go through during a sexual encounter. Some people go through them quickly and are ready for sex at the drop of a hat, while others are slow starts and might need 15 minutes of foreplay to truly get into the mood.

The same variance applies to the types of dirty talk that

people like. Some like it sweet, and some like it rough. Some might feel degraded, and some might want more degrading. Some want to be your slave, and some want to dominate you with a choke collar. There's nothing wrong with any of those – the only wrong thing is if you don't figure out which style works best for you and your partner.

It's up to you to discover you and your partner's optimal blend of dirty talk, and the easiest way to do so is to use a wide variety of dirty talk phrases and pay attention to your partner's verbal and non-verbal response. That will help you determine what really makes sparks fly, and what your go-tos should be.

Be careful with degrading dirty talk, as it has been shown to sometimes make women feel more emotionally distant from their partners, which is of course the opposite effect you want to have.

A final important part of calibrating to your partner is having a post-mortem discussion about what went well, what you each liked, and what should never be used again. Unsurprisingly, communication is key!

### *Just moan, damnit*

If you're having sex right, sometimes you won't have a clear enough head to even form words in your mind.

So in lieu of dirty talk, oftentimes you should make an effort to moan and react effectively to your partner's actions. Any type of vocalization is going to enhance the experience, and sometimes a primal series of moans and whimpers can get the point across more succinctly and clearly than a well-placed "I want you inside of me."

Focusing on reacting will make you more present and in the moment with the experience, while some dirty talk practitioners can become slightly distant because they are focused on thinking about the next phrase to whisper.

Again, this is a good intermediate step for beginners to small talk. Simply breaking the sound barrier can be transformative, and moans and groans are easier to let slip and test the waters than dirty talk.

Finally, as I mentioned before, you don't actually have to respond to the questions that your partner might ask you during dirty talk.

*"You like that?" "Why, yes, I enjoy it very much, thanks."*

A lot of them are rhetorical in nature, and don't need a response for the intended effect. But you could always moan in acknowledgement, which would be a good way to get your feet wet, as well as show your appreciation of their dirty talk.

And now, finally what you've been waiting for. When most people want to learn about dirty talk, I find that they usually just want exact creative and sexy phrases that they can borrow. I have no problem with this, as I've learned many phrases from others as well.

We all need a baseline to start with before we can really discover our true dirty talk personality and character.

### General guidelines

1. Describe how they are making you feel by what they are doing to you in that moment. Make it personal, that they are the ones affecting you and only them.
2. Direct them — command, ask, beg, demand, or plead. Also, add "please" to many dirty talk phrases.
3. Narrate your actions. Tell them what you are doing, or what you are going to do to them.
4. Praise them. Be specific, and focus on their physical attributes. Many people's self-esteem is wrapped up in their physical appearance, so if you praise them, you are simultaneously building their confidence as well as dirty talking. When someone is more confident about their body and has high self-esteem, they'll be more likely to explore new thing and be open — this can only work in your favor.
5. Talk in terms of possessions. You are hers, she is yours. Your cock is hers, her pussy is yours. Etc.
6. You don't have to actually answer a question they pose in their dirty talk. Many are rhetorical. As long as you acknowledge it or even moan to it, that is sufficient.

As you'll see, these six guidelines will be present in almost of all the dirty talk phrases I give you in this book.

For ease of digestion and visualization, I've grouped my dirty talk phrases into a few distinct phases. They run the gamut of when you could use them related to a sexual encounter, from days to weeks of teasing, to the actual encounter, during the orgasm, and afterwards. I'll educate you on the goals and tones you should be using for each phase.

Most of these phrases are fairly unisex and can be used without regard to gender or sexual orientation... and they are easily altered to fit your needs otherwise.

### Setting the stage

This is the phase before you even see your paramour. This might be through texting, emailing, chatting, or even over the phone. The point here is to drive anticipation and hint at the promise of what's to come later. You can do this throughout the day, or week even, to make them hunger for you. The trick in setting the stage is to talk in future terms of what you want them to do to you, and what you want to do to them.

Have the mindset of trying to lure your partner over immediately – what would you say to tempt them? Imagine getting a text or email like this at work and the hungry reaction that you'll create.
1.  I want you so bad

2. God I miss feeling you

3. You are going to feel so good inside me

4. I miss feeling your cock/pussy

5. I want you to lick my cock/pussy right now

6. I am going to pound you raw

7. I am going to drink all of your cum

8. I can't get enough of you

9. I need to taste you right now

10. I'm hard/wet just thinking about you

11. You make me so hard/wet

12. You drive me crazy

13. I dreamt about fucking you last night

14. I can't wait for you to spread me

15. I can't wait to spread you

16. I can't wait to fuck you from behind

17. I can't stop thinking about how you moan

18. I can't stop thinking about your pussy/cock

19. I am going to fill you up with my cum

20. How do you want to fuck me on Saturday?

21. How much cum are you going to give me on Saturday?

22. I don't want to wait for your cock/pussy

23. Only you can fuck me right

24. My pussy/cock aches for you

25. Tell me how you're going to fuck me

26. Fuck me please?

27. You're the tightest/biggest

28. I want to taste you now.

29. I love how you look at me when we fuck

30. Your pussy/cock is mine

## Foreplay

For the purposes of this book, I'm counting foreplay as the moment your lips meet, and including everything until actual penetration. This includes oral and manual stimulation. Foreplay is all about teasing and increasing the anticipation for the main event. Focus on your partner and how they are making you feel, while hinting that the main event is going to blow your mind because of the anticipation you've had.

Have the mindset that you are in the desert and they are your oasis – you just can't get enough of them, and they can do no wrong. Make them feel amazing about themselves, and they will want to reciprocate physically.

1. You feel so good

2. Your smell is intoxicating

3. You feel amazing

4. You're so sexy/hot

5. I could do this all day

6. I love when you [fill in the blank]

7. Your skin feels so good

8. Your lips are so soft

9. Bite me

10. Spank my ass

11. Use your nails on me

12. Feel how hard/wet you make me

13. Just looking at you makes me hard/wet

14. You drive me crazy

15. Fuck my face

16. Strip now

17. Pull my hair

18. Dominate me

19. What do you want me to do?

20. Lie back, it's my turn

21. You look so hot sucking my cock

22. I want you in my mouth

23. You're so tight

24. You taste so good/sweet

25. You're so hard

26. Your pussy/cock tastes so good

27. Shove your tongue in me

28. Grab my cock and play with my balls

29. Tell me what to do

30. Gag on it

31. Make me gag

32. Rub your clit now

33. Can I put your cock in my mouth please?

34. Do you like that?

35. You have a nice load in there for me? [while grabbing

    his cock]

36. Everything about you turns me on

37. Kiss/suck my cock/pussy/clit

38. Your pussy/cock is mine

39. My cock/pussy is yours.

40. Am I being a good/bad girl?

41. Make me beg

42. Tease me

43. Don't tease me, just do it

44. You can have anything you want

45. Feel how ready I am [take his/her hand and lead it to your genitals]

46. You want to fuck me, don't you

47. Wrap your legs around me

48. You want to feel my cock in you?

49. I can't wait to be inside you

50. I need you inside me

51. Please?

## Intercourse

Of course, intercourse counts as any form of penetration. Since this is the main event, talk about how you've waited eagerly for this, and that it's living up to all of your expectations. Talk about the actual thrusting and the mechanics that you enjoy behind it. Talk about how passionately you want the sex to be.

Try having the mindset that every thrust is mind-blowing, and that you can barely stop from orgasming from their touch. It's not true of course, but projecting such passion will turn your partner into an echo chamber.

1. Don't stop pounding me

2. Make me scream

3. Your pussy is so warm/tight

4. Your cock is so hot/big

5. You're filling me up

6. Fuck me harder

7. You feel so tight

8. Right there

9. Deeper

10. Only you can fuck me like this

11. Only you know how I love it

12. Give me that cock/pussy

13. I'm going to fuck you until you break

14. May I come?

15. You make me feel so full

16. Fuck that feels so good

17. That cock feels so good in my pussy

18. That's my good/bad girl

19. Say my name

20. Flip over and spread your pussy

21. Look at me

22. You look amazing spread under me/bent over

23. Choke me

24. I love feeling you inside me

25. Do you like that?

26. You are so hot

27. You drive me wild

28. I want to make you cum

29. Make me cum

30. I'm going to watch you cum

31. You're so deep

32. Do you like it deep?

33. I need you

34. I've been thinking about this all day

35. You're going to make me cum so hard

36. You like when I spread for you?

37. I'm going to suck you until you come

38. Ride me harder

39. You're my naughty girl

40. Bend over, slut

41. I love fucking you

42. Lick it clean

43. I'm going to clean you clean

44. You're so hard inside me

45. Moan for me

46. You're driving me crazy

47. I'm going to fuck you until you can't walk

48. I'm so fucking wet

49. Beg me

50. You own me

51. Take it all

52. You're my fucktoy now

53. Make me your fucktoy

54. You can do anything you want to me

55. Fuck my cunt

56. Spread your pussy lips

57. Tell me what you want

58. You're making me shake

59. Fuck me raw

60. Fuck me from behind

61. Make it hurt

62. Do you have any idea what you're doing to me?

63. I love your [fill in the blank]

## *Orgasm*

This is where it's all been leading to. This is where you find your sense of relief, and the culmination of everything you've anticipated of your partner. Express it! Talk about how long you've wanted this, and that your partner is so irresistible that you simply couldn't help yourself. Cumplay is a big fetish for both genders, so having it inside, outside, on the woman's chest, in the mans' hair – someone is going to thoroughly it any way you do it.

Your mindset here should be that your orgasm is from your partner, by your partner, and solely for your partner.

1. I'm going to fill you up

2. Fill me up

3. I'm coming

4. Don't stop until you're empty

5. Come all over my cock

6. Take every drop

7. I'm coming all over your cock

8. I can't hold back any longer

9. I can't resist your cock/pussy

10. I can't take it anymore

11. Don't stop until I cum

12. You're going to make me cum

13. Give me your cum

14. Never stop, don't stop

15. I want to watch you come

16. Let's come together

17. Watch me cum for you

18. Can I come sir?

19. Watch me come for you

20. Come for me

21. Make me drip

22. Come in my mouth

23. I can't stop coming for you

24. Take it all

25. Look what you're doing to me

26. Shoot it deep inside me

27. I want to swallow you

28. Make my pussy scream

29. Where do you want me to come?

30. Come inside me

## Post-coital

This is the phase after you catch your breath from the amazing orgasm that you just had due to your newfound dirty talk skills. They've heightened your experience and left you a sweaty mess. All you can do now is lament that it was over too soon, and look to setting the tone for the next session. Take this opportunity to praise your partner, talk about what you loved about the experience you just shared, and what you are looking forward to for the next one.

Your mindset here should be that you're sad that it was over so soon, but despite that, you can barely move from the orgasm.

1. You're so amazing/That was amazing

2. You're mine

3. I'm yours

4. Look what you did to me

5. I can't help myself around you

6. We're going to go again in 5 minutes

7. Make me beg for more

8. I can't control myself around you

9. How did you do that?

10. Next time, you can do whatever you want to me

11. You look so good full of my cum

12. I love you freshly fucked

13. I'm your toy, do whatever you want to me

14. I've been thinking about that for days

15. How long until you're ready for round 2?

16. Don't make me wait to fuck me again

17. You made me shake

18. You made me numb

19. Oh my God... (keep repeating this)

20. I need more of you

21. I love fucking/pounding you

22. Let me lick you clean

23. I can't feel my toes

24. You made me come so hard I'm shaking

25. Only you can fuck me so good

26. Your pussy/cock is amazing

27. Did you like being fucking used (like a fucktoy)?

28. You broke me

29. I'm going to be sore tomorrow

30. You're the best I've ever had

## 5. Mastering real foreplay.

In the previous chapter, I talked about the emotional and psychological layers of foreplay. If you want to master foreplay, you need to master how to get your female partner excited on an emotional and psychological level before physical sex.

With that said, this chapter is devoted to physical foreplay.

Setting the mood and environment.

As I've mentioned in an earlier chapter, women look at sex primarily focused on comfort, security, and trust. You are communicating to your partner that you get this when you set the right mood and environment. Setting the right mood as far as physical foreplay is concerned is all about setting the right environment.

Make sure that the lighting is right, the temperature is just right, and that physically, the environment is there to calm her down and set her at ease.

Does this mean you can't have hot, sweaty, and monkey sex in a very hot area or out in the rain? Absolutely not. It happens all the time. All I'm saying is that if you want to be the master of foreplay, you may want to play it conventionally and this is the way to do it by taking care of setting the right mood and environment first. Make her comfortable, and make sure your bedroom and bathroom has all the requisite amenities.

Hygiene.

I don't know why I'm even saying this, but you'd be surprised as to how uncommon common sense is in this modern day and age. You have to take care of hygiene.

Unless your woman is into five-o-clock shadows and beards, you might want to shave. You might want to take a shower first and smell pleasant. You might want to be clean and not have any dirt marks over you. You might want to cut your nails.

Hygiene is one of the signals you're sending out to your partner. The whole point of hygiene is to make sure that you're not doing anything or not appearing like something that would get in the way of your partner getting in the right mood. This sets the groundwork for real foreplay.

Play with her breasts.

The breast has actually many different zones. Most guys would just go straight to the nipple and start sucking on it. This is perfectly understandable, but the breast actually has many different zones, and you need to play the zones.

You need to go through the steps to play the zones in sequence.

Start with the sides of the breast and then work your way to the front massage the sides of the nipples. At this point, you can do many different things. You can lick the nipple and around the areola. This has nerve endings that are quite sensitive. However, those nerve endings really build-up in sensitivity when you massage the sides of the breast first. Remember, when it comes to tit play, sequence is everything.

Also, you might want to play it like a Jedi master and breathe on them a little bit, blow on them, tickle them with the tip of your tongue. Also, make eye contact when you are doing breast play. It shows her that you treasure her, that you prize her, and this is all about you and her.

Kissing.

When you kiss a woman, you have to build it up properly. You have to first start with the edges of the lips, and you might want to suck the edges of her lips into yours. This expresses your excitement in wanting her, but you don't want to overdo it and vacuum her lips into your mouth.

Depending on how heated she is, maybe this is what exactly needs to happen, but you have to play it by ear. If you're just starting it out, you need to build it up softly, but once you are already fucking her, it's perfectly okay to just suck her face in because the intensity is already there. If you're just beginning, you might want to dial it down.

With kissing, start at the edges of the lips. You might want to softly bite down and then work your tongue into her mouth. First, touch the tip of her tongue and then as things heat it up, explore the rest of her tongue and a little bit of inside of her mouth.

The whole point of French kissing is to show passion and intensity. You're basically penetrating her mouth with your tongue.

You cannot just jam your tongue into her. Again, this would be perfectly acceptable if you're already penetrating her down below. That's always a good move when you have her in doggie style. She might feel isolated if you're just minding your own business behind her. I hope you see the point.

Biting and nibbling.

The back of the ear is very sensitive. Also, when you have a tongue in your ear, it's very sensitive so use this to your advantage. Breath into her ear and lick at the same time.

Nibble at her earlobes. Nibble at the backside of her neck near her ear and then gently bite.

We're not talking about vampire bites. You gently bite meaning cushion your bite with your tongue or your lips enough to make her feel the pressure but not enough to leave her a mark.

A little spanking.

Spanking is great when the woman assumes a position on top of you during foreplay. You might want to spank her a little bit on her butt. Some guys screw up and slap the back of her thigh. That's painful especially is she has her pants off. So the whole point of spanking is again to send a physical message that you desire and want her and physically signal that you're going to be penetrating soon.

Hair pulling.

Some women like to have their head yanked back and like sex to be very physical and forceful. They like to be taken. However, you cannot assume that all women are like this so you need to gently pull her hair back. If you detect any sort of resistance, you need to let go. You don't want to kill the mood with a bad move or misjudgment on your part.

So if you're going to do a little bit of hair pulling, make sure it's gentle and you escalate it slowly because you might be with a girl who is very big on hair pulling, likes a tongue jammed down her throat, a little bit of rough spanking, and just basically feeling like she's being taken.

However, in all likelihood, you are probably with a woman who wants something much less than that so let her lead the way. You can suggest through gently hair pulling and slight escalation. If she resists, then that's your cue to let go.

Pro tip: grab the hair at the base of the skull, which puts less pressure on each individual hair strand and makes it much more pleasurable for her in general.

Fingering.

Guys really drop the ball when it comes to inserting their fingers up a woman's vagina. Fingering is an art form. You can't just jam your finger up there. You're not doing a gynecological exam and you're not her OB-Gyn.

You have to first massage the area. We're talking of course about clitoral stimulation. At the top of the vaginal opening is this little hooded part called the clitoris. It's kind of like there's a hood of flesh and when you pull it back, there's a little button. You might want to gently rub it with your thumb. The keyword here is gently.

When you notice some changes in her behavior like she puts her hand on top of your hand and pushes your hand to move it faster, that's your cue. Rub her clitoris faster and harder but don't over do it. You don't want to rub it raw. Again, she's not a guy. Guys stimulate themselves by just simply moving faster and increasing intensity. Women don't work that way.

The next step is then to rub your thumb and index finger around the sides of her vaginal lips and then slowly work your way one finger at a time into her vagina.

CAUTION: Make sure that her pussy is wet, and literally glistening with moisture. If it's not, then your fingers will actually hurt her. Imagine sandpaper on your penis. That's the feeling. So you have to make sure that she is turned on enough and wet enough for this step.

Guys think that as long they just have two fingers inside a woman's pussy, they're doing a good job. I'm sorry to say, but you're not doing the job right if you think you're doing okay just by having your fingers up her. It doesn't that work way. You have to explore the space.

When you have your index finger in her, point up and then try to point back towards your body, you would see that there's an area that appears to have ridges and feels like the outside of a walnut.

This is the G-spot. The G-spot is never the same with the same woman and definitely among different women. It's your job to look for it, and you will notice that you've found it based on how much she moans, how much she moves around, and how she bucks against your hand.

If you continue that motion of making a "come here" sign with your finger(s) against the G-spot, you can induce a G-spot orgasm, which is a form of a vaginal orgasm. It requires a good amount of speed and intensity for most women.

## 6. The inside scoop on oral sex.

Just like with anything else sexual, you have to understand that sex is primarily a psychological state. I know this is going to come off as a shock to most guys because most of us think that sex is primarily biological: part A going into part B.

If you want to orally please your woman, you have to understand how first sending the right emotional signals and setting up the right psychological tone can lead to a more fulfilling and rewarding time for her.

Tease her properly.

The best way to go down on a woman is not just to open your mouth and jam your tongue right up her pussy. Again, while some chicks dig this, most don't.

You have to send a signal to her that you are going down that way. Maybe you would want to nibble on her tits first, massage the side of her breast, and then lick her tummy.

This buildup psychologically prepares her for the fact that you are going to be putting your head between her legs. The way you do it is also very important. You can't just do this mechanically like you're going through a checklist, or you are painting by numbers. That pretty much strips all the soul out of great oral sex.

You have to tease her a bit. Look into her eyes. Have a smile in your eyes and then close your eyes, so there's a bit of mystery. You need to tickle the back of her ears, stimulate the side of her breasts while you're moving your tongue down her body.

Teasing is a very important part of any kind of sex act. It sends a signal to your partner that you're about to do something. It also increases the receptivity of their nerves. You want to reduce your partner into this quivering and highly excited mass of nerves. The more excited she gets, the easier it is for her to cum.

Clitoral stimulation.

The secret to clitoral stimulation is that you need to treat her like the way your woman treats your penis when she's blowing it. Seriously. You have to treat it like a small version of your penis. So you need to tease it, suck on it, blow on it, and then you need to move your jaw while you're doing it.

Nothing is more boring than just simply licking a clitoris.

Chances are your woman has been around the block a couple of times. She's probably been with at least one other guy, and this is not a completely new experience to her. You have to demonstrate to her that you know how to stimulate a clitoris properly, and this means you need to move your jaw. There has to be some sort of motion there. It's not just your tongue moving. It's also your jaw, which makes your tongue motions stronger and more vigorous.

Also, you need to make an "o" with your mouth and suck up the clitoris and then lick it slowly. While you're doing this, you need to be doing things with your hands. You can be looking for that G-spot while you are licking her clitoris, holding her hips down, spreading her legs, massaging her breasts, or even playing with her anus.

Try to stay away from simply licking. You also need to blow, tease - this means touching the tip of her clitoris with the tip of your tongue, and pinching LIGHTLY with your lips.

You have to exercise a lot of variety when you are engaging her clitoris. Otherwise, it's going to be boring, and the sensation would really not be much different from that produced by a vibrator. If a machine can do your job, then your woman doesn't need you.

So do a better job and this means putting her needs ahead of yours in giving oral foreplay the amount of time and energy and passion it deserves.

Finally, make it wet. Use lots of saliva, and don't be afraid of getting messy and slobbering. This will enhance all the sensations, and dryness on her pussy is just unpleasant and sometimes painful. This also gives the appearance of passion, which will turn her on by how into oral sex you are.

Techniques and positions.

When it comes to oral stimulation, the best technique would be for her to be comfortable so that she can tune everything else out and just focus on the sensations that you are giving her.

It takes a long time for women to get excited and takes an even longer time for them to cum. You have to position her body so she can reach that point all while remaining comfortable.

The classic position is for her to be on her back with her legs spread. This allows easy access to her breasts, and is comfortable for her.

Another position is for her to sit on your face. You lie on your back and literally pull her on top of you so that her pussy in over your mouth. This can be erotic as she can control the speed and intensity of the oral sex more than she would be able to otherwise.

Finally, I'm a big fan of the woman being on her hands and knees, and you licking her pussy from behind her. This is less comfortable for both of you, but as a short interlude between sex positions, it can be extremely arousing to see her from this position.

So how do you know you did the job right? She came.

## 7. The not-so-fun chapter.

In the previous chapters of this book, I have gone through the fun stuff.

I have helped you get inside the head of a typical woman. I've helped you understand why men and women respond to sex differently.

I have also stepped you through the process of mental, emotional, and physical foreplay. We have even talked about oral sex.

Now comes the not-so-fun part. We are talking about stuff that you need to take care of before you engage in sex.

Usually this should go before foreplay. Before any kind of physical contact, you should have this squared away. But, I figured I would put this before the chapter on penetration, for emphasis.

There is a lot of not-so-fun stuff that you need to focus on, before you get down and dirty. If you don't take care of this checklist of items, you might end up in all sorts of trouble.

At the very least, you might get sick. At the very worst, you might end up dead in a ditch somewhere.

Birth control.

You have to be responsible when it comes to birth control. You don't want the couple of hours of fun you spend with your partner to lead to 18 years of mandatory child support. In the United States, if you get a woman pregnant and she gets a court order, you are on the hook, financially, for 18 years. There are exceptions, but don't consider that your backup plan.

Every time you get a paycheck, a chunk of that paycheck goes automatically to your baby mama. If you don't want that to happen, you need to wrap it up... otherwise that is the most expensive sex you've ever had.

Now, most guys think that, as long as they put on a rubber, they are good to go. Well, wrapping up is just the first part of the equation. Simply putting a condom on is just taking care of 80% of the picture. What about the 20%?

You have to remember that condoms break. You have to remember that, depending on the size of your equipment, and how tight your partner is, condoms slip off. That is just the fact of life.

You need to cover all your bases. I highly suggest that you also use spermicidal lube. There are all sorts of products on the market that will not only lubricate your junk, but also kill of any of your little guys that make it out. This way, even if you spill, you can rest assured that your partner won't get pregnant.

Ideally, your partner should also be on some contraception as well. Ideally, she should be on the pill, and you should find out before the deed so you can know if you are double protected, or only single with a condom.

Regardless, you need to think about birth control before you have sex.

Sexually transmitted diseases.

Sexually Transmitted Diseases are a fact of life.

The worst part of this is that there are certain STDs, like Chlamydia, that are often asymptomatic. You might be banging this hot beach bunny who looks extremely healthy and athletic, but she is supporting Chlamydia.

How bad can Chlamydia get? Well, let's put it this way. Once you reach that point in your life when you want to have kids, you can no longer have kids. That is how bad Chlamydia is. It can strip out your reproductive capabilities and make you infertile. Chlamydia is particularly deadly to the reproductive system of females.

Be on the lookout for STDs. Even with treatable and curable diseases like Syphilis and Gonorrhea, you really can't let your guard down. Why? There are many resistant strains of Syphilis and Gonorrhea going around. This means that the typical cocktail of antibiotics no longer work on them.

At the very least, you need to use a condom. But you need to go further than a condom. You have to remember that Herpes can be spread even if you are wearing a condom.

The big step here is to make sure that you yourself are checked out every couple of months (more or less, depending on just how many new partners you're having), and talk to your potential partner about the last time they got tested before the act. It's a difficult conversation, but is sex worth a bunch of blisters and sores on your penis? Probably not.

Consent and rape issues.

It is very easy for guys to think that the woman is very willing.

Really, you would be surprised as to the kinds of tricks our minds play on us, especially if we are hot, horny, and bothered. But if you think for a second that the woman you are with hasn't given you full consent, or is resistant, stop what you are doing. That is rape.

Determine whether her "no" is really a "NO!"

Also, if she is asleep, or she is stoned or drunk, don't do it. According to the law, if somebody is asleep, drunk, drugged out, or otherwise incapacitated - we are talking about low IQ and mentally incapacitated as well - you cannot legally have sex with that person. Why? They do not have the right, under the law, to give you consent.

The big difference between rape and regular sex is consent. If the woman doesn't give you consent, you are raping her. You can go to jail. There is no way to dance around this, so make sure you get consent. As much as possible, make her say it, "I want you to fuck me." Or make her say something to that effect.

Rape and consent issues get a little blurrier when you factor in rough sex, rape play, slapping, choking, and any number of kinks that women might have. A good rule of thumb is simply ask (in a way that doesn't kill the mood) whether they want to be slapped in the face, and make sure her answer is a clear yes.

## 7.5. A peak into exactly what turns a woman on…

We have talked a little bit about how different men and women are – it is biological at the very least.

What turns you on will be very different from what turns a woman on, and that is illustrated very clearly by the popularity of erotica and romance novels.

Guess who reads erotica and romance? 95% of the consumers are women. Where men might prefer something visual, a woman will prefer something sensual, romantic, and left to the imagination.

Just take a peak at at the following romance novel that has proven extremely popular with women and see firsthand what turns them on. Note the buildup, anticipation, vocabulary, and how the men act in the novel to the women. The men are dominant, strong, sensitive, and caring. That should be your rule of thumb.

I repeat – look at how much background, context, and buildup there is. Realize how mental sex can be for women! There are only three sex scenes in the following book, so what fills the rest of the pages? Story, romance, anticipation, description, and character backstories. Certainly something to think about.

By the way, if you want to just skip to the sex scenes, go to pages 105, 117, and 140. I wouldn't blame you.

## Seduced By The Badass – a taboo romance story

**Chapter 1**

The night was heavy with the perfume of freshly mown grass and the promise of summer rain. Lois Carmody breathed it in as she stared out her bedroom window. The heat of the day had been almost unbearable and because the broken air conditioner, inescapable. Lois appreciated the breeze that had finally begun to blow, and she had opened her bedroom window to welcome it in.

She sat in her bra and panties, unwilling to dress in anything else because of the heat. Her bedroom door stood open, but she knew no one could see her in the darkness. No moon shone through the clouds above, nor did any streetlights shine below. She was confident of the privacy offered by her step-father's home.

The lake house was located in Hunt's Point, a wealthy suburb of Seattle, Washington. The town was situated on a peninsula, surrounded by Lake Washington. It was a beautiful place.

Frogs croaked and crickets chirped, filling the night with sweet music. The breeze shifted, and Lois now smelled the lake along with the other mélange of scents. She smiled.

Though they were experiencing an unusual heat wave, this place was a far cry from Los Angeles, the city where she and her sister Mabel had grown up. She had always been sick there, unable to adapt to the poisonous concoction of carbon monoxide and civilization. Her mother's marriage to Tim O'Reilly had been a true blessing. It had taken them almost overnight from a life of poverty and delivered them to one of luxury. Sometimes, she believed the move had saved her life.

A soft knock sounded on her door. Mabel stood in the doorway.

"Are you still awake?" Mabel asked. "I thought you'd be exhausted after all that swimming today."
"Too hot," Lois replied.

Mabel walked in, closed the door part-way and switched on the bedside lamp. The soft glow of an energy saver bulb lit the room and revealed the pink, baby-doll nightie her sister wore. Lois frowned. "Does Mom know you've got that?"

Mabel grinned. "Like it? I got it at the mall the other

day." She twirled around. The nightie barely covered the matching G-string. "And, yes, Mom knows. She said to pick out anything I wanted for my birthday and this was it."

Lois shook her head. "You're only seventeen..."
"And I'll be eighteen on Saturday. Stop being such an old fogey! Geez! I swear ever since Mom got married, you've been a huge party pooper. Lighten up!" She punctuated her statement by jumping onto the end of Lois's waterbed.

"Knock it off!" Lois cried. "You know I hate that!"
Mabel crossed her legs and arranged the nightie over her lap. "Are you coming to my slumber party?"
"You know you're too old for a slumber party," Lois said. "Why in the world did you talk Mom into letting you have one?"

"Good grief, Lois! I'm too young for this baby-doll, but too old for a slumber party? How old do I have to act before you stop hounding me?"
"I'm sorry. I didn't mean to sound that way. It's just been so hot today."

"Speaking of hot," Mabel said, her brown eyes sparkling with mischief, "Guess who's coming to the party. I'll give you a hint. It's not a girl..."
"You can't have guys at your slumber party!" Lois said. "Mom would never allow that. Even Tim would put his foot down on that one."

"I happen to know that he will be most welcome. After all, he already lives here."

Lois's eyes widened. "You're inviting Seamus to the party?"

"Well, not in so many words, but I'm sure I can convince him to stay home that day. Maybe, I'll even give him a little preview of what I'll be wearing."

"That's disgusting!" Lois crinkled her nose. "He's our step-brother."

"Step-brothers are, by definition, unrelated. As far as I am concerned, he's fair game. Besides, I saw you drooling over him today. So don't tell me you don't think he's hot."

Lois froze. Had it really been that obvious? She shook her head in denial. "He's not my type," she insisted, hoping her sister would believe her. "Or yours either."

"Oh, that's right! Miss Goody-Two-Shoes would never be seen with a convict."

"A convict! Is that where he's been for the last three years? Prison?"

"I'd say so. Did you see all of his tattoos and the way he's beefed up? He didn't have muscles like that when he was 17."

"That doesn't mean anything. Everybody has tattoos now. Did he say he'd been in prison?"

"He hasn't said anything about where he's been. I'm

just glad Tim let him come back. After the fight they had, I thought he'd be disowned."

Lois nodded. She remembered that altercation. It had raised the roof off the house. Tim O'Reilly was a stubborn, full-blooded Irishman who loved a good fight and his son was no different. She didn't know what, exactly, they had fought about, but it had certainly put them at odds with each other. Watching them that night, they'd reminded her of two rams butting heads.

Of course, at that time, Seamus had been mostly out of control. He and his father hadn't really gotten along for several years. It all stemmed back to Seamus's childhood.

When Seamus had been born, his father had been a part-owner of a construction company. He hadn't been home much and, while he was gone, his wife had gotten involved with another man. One day, while Seamus had been at school, Tim had come home to find the house empty. His wife, Kris, had left with her lover.

She had had no interest in her son until four years later, when his father had become wealthy. Perhaps her bid for custody and support would have been more successful if she hadn't been forced into drug rehab.

Tim had been fair to his ex-wife. He had taken custody of Seamus, but had allowed her visitation. During the summers the boy would live with Kris in Anaheim. The rest of the year, he would reside with his father in Los Angeles. The custody agreement had gone into effect as soon as Kris had been judged clean and sober. The first summer had gone well and Seamus had seemed to rebuild his relationship with his mother. He would talk to her daily and would send her letters and pictures through e-mail. The next summer, though, things had gone downhill.

Tim had been in a business meeting, when he had received an emergency phone call from his son. Seamus had begged his father to come and pick him up from his mother's. He had claimed that his vacation with her was done. Tim had left his important meeting in a rush and had driven the twenty-six miles to Anaheim.

When Tim had arrived at the house in Anaheim, Seamus had been playing video games. Nothing had seemed. He had left without Seamus, feeling very foolish.

This same incident had been repeated three more times. Finally, Tim became tired of "the boy who cried wolf" scenario, and the next time Seamus had called for help, he didn't go to Anaheim.

Lois had overheard Tim telling her mother this story

the night of the big fight. It had been shortly after that when Seamus had stormed out, vowing never to return. She'd missed the last part of the story because Mabel had come to sleep with her in her room.

Consequently, Lois had no idea what had happened to Seamus that summer. All she knew was that Seamus never went back to stay with his mother and somehow blamed his father for whatever had happened.

Tim had become involved with their mother, Cathy, six years later. By then, Seamus had been well on his way to becoming a juvenile delinquent. He had been smoking, drinking and fighting and had become an embarrassment to his father.

But to Lois, then a girl of seventeen, Seamus had been fascinating. At that time, he had been thinner, with black hair and piercing blue eyes. He was only a few months older than her, and back then they had often found things to talk about. She had felt, at one time, that they were friends.

Lois's recalled one of her favorite memories, when Seamus had been standing outside near a friend's motorcycle, wearing a black leather jacket. The collar had been turned up and he had glanced up at her as she stood by her bedroom window and winked.
Her worst memory was the Senior Prom. He had taken a popular girl, Denise Allen, and they had ended

up having sex in the Ladies Room. Lois had walked in on them and had been utterly humiliated. The only good part about that memory was that she had actually seen him naked for the first time.

Even now, she got a little chill when she thought about it.

The bathroom door had had an "Out of Order" sign on it, but Lois had needed to go in the worst way. She had slipped in, hoping to make a quick pit stop, but then she had heard moans echoing in the tiled room. The bathroom had been designed for privacy and she had had to walk around a corner before entering the main room itself. When she had rounded that corner, she had found them.

She had barely noticed Denise, who had been leaning against the sink, facing the mirror. All Lois had seen was Seamus.  His muscles had been taught and well-defined. One hand had clutched Denise's left breast while the other had clasped her right hip. His long legs had been spread a little while he took her from behind. He had looked up in surprise when she had walked in, his dark hair plastered to his forehead. On anyone else, it might have looked terribly unappealing, even comical. To her, though, it had only added to Seamus's attractiveness. When he had seen her staring at him, he had pulled out of Denise. At that point, Denise had noticed her as well, and she'd given a little cry as she scrambled into a stall to hide. Lois had hardly paid any attention.  Her eyes had been fixed to Seamus's nether regions.

His had been the first penis she had ever seen, and it had been superb.

She still remembered how swollen and pink had been, even in those dreadful fluorescent lights. She had marveled at it, wondering what such a thing would feel like inside. When she had finally looked up, she had realized that he had been watching her intently. A crimson flush had risen over the collar of her modest Prom dress and had crept across her face. She had dashed from the room.

The moment had brought to the surface feelings she hadn't known existed.  She had never told anyone about what she'd seen.

That had happened back in Los Angeles, a few years before their move to Cathy's home in Washington. Lois remembered it as though it were yesterday.

It had been hard to be around Seamus after that. She had avoided him at the house for a while. She needn't have worried though. A few days later, he had the argument that sent him away for three long years and had forced him to miss his graduation.

Now, he was back. And he was sexier than ever.

"Earth to Lois! Come back, Lois!" Mabel was saying, her hands cupped over her mouth.

Lois returned to the present. "I'm sorry, what did you say?"

"I said, Tim's going to give Seamus a job. Something in the construction company. He'll be hanging around here a lot more. At least until he gets his own place."
"Is that another rumor?" Lois asked. "Or do you know it for a fact."

"It's a fact. I heard Tim telling Mom."
A knot formed in Lois's stomach.
"Well, I still doubt that he'll be at your slumber party. It would be pretty weird for a 20 year-old guy to be hanging out with teenage girls."

"I didn't say he'd be hanging out with them. I said he'd be hanging out with me."
"You're so gross," she said, scowling.
"You're just jealous."

"No, I'm in control of my hormones. Unlike you."
"Who's not in control of their hormones?" a voice said from the hallway. The voice was deep, velvety. Lois's lips suddenly went dry as the door opened on silent hinges. Seamus stood in the doorway, leaning against it.

He wore no shirt, just jeans. His feet were bare. Tattoos sleeved both arms. The illustrations were vibrant against his tanned skin. The one that caught Lois's eye was the topless woman on the back of his forearm. Her breasts were large and a little too realistic in appearance. As Mabel had said, he did look beefed up. His muscles were nothing, however, compared to his twinkling blue eyes and mane of black hair. They made her weak in the knees.

"Apparently, I am," Mabel said. She had turned and was trying to get off the bed, when Lois caught her by the arm and pulled her back.
"There is no way you're showing him that G-string in my room!" she hissed.

"At least I have a nightie on. You're in your underwear." Mabel whispered back.
Seamus's eyes seemed to express his approval at her state of undress. There was a comforter at the end of the bed and she snatched it up. He looked mildly disappointed when she covered herself, or at least she thought he did.

"Were your ears burning, Seamus?" Mabel asked.
"We were talking about you."
"You were?" His voice was smooth, exuding a dream-like quality. Lois had always loved the sound of it. He entered the room and closed the door. Her heart quickened.

"What's the matter, Lois?" he asked. "You look like a deer caught in the headlights. I've been in your room plenty of times before."
That was before I saw you naked, she thought to herself.

"Oh, don't pay attention to the party pooper here," Mabel said. "Speaking of parties..."

"Yes?"

"Are you coming to mine?"

He eyed her intently. Mabel smiled under his scrutiny.

"Maybe," he said.

"Good," Mabel replied.

She's acting as though he agreed to come! Lois fumed. "Maybe he'll be busy that night." she said, looking up at him, her eyes disapproving. He seemed amused by her expression.

"I could be," he said with a nod.

"Awww!" Mabel pouted. "I haven't seen you in three years and you won't even come to my birthday party?" Tears appeared in her eyes as though on command.

"Well, how can I refuse that?" Seamus said. "I can't stay away from my favorite step-sister's party."

Mabel squealed and leaped off the bed. She threw her arms around his neck and shamelessly pressed herself against him. He patted her on the back.

Lois remained underneath the comforter. A sheen of sweat covered her skin. She felt a little sick.

"I'm so glad!" Mabel kissed Seamus on the cheek.

Lois's narrowed her eyes.

"It's so good to have you back!" Mabel gushed.

"Good to be back," Seamus said with smile.

"I think you should both go to bed now," Lois said to Mabel.

"That's a good idea," Mabel said. Her voice low and almost husky. With the pretense of saying goodnight to Lois, she turned around. Her action ensured that Seamus received a generous view of her new underwear.

"Goodnight, Lois," Mabel said. Her smile was wicked.

"Goodnight, Mabel," she replied. The girl was incorrigible.

Mabel turned and smiled at Seamus. Then she opened the door and trotted out of the room.

Seamus didn't leave the room. To Lois's dismay, he took a seat in the room's only chair. He straddled it, resting his arms on the back. The busty woman on his arm stared at her.

"What about you, Lois? Are you glad to see me back?" his tone was neutral, but she detected a hint of nervousness in it.

"I'm glad you're back. It wasn't the same without you around." She pulled the comforter up until it touched her chin.

"Aren't you kind of hot under that?" he asked.

"No, I'm fine." Sweat trickled down her belly. She shifted uncomfortably.

"I gotta say, I'm surprised you're still here. I thought

you'd have gone to college, or gotten married."
"Me? Married? I don't even have a boyfriend. As to college, well, I tried it. It didn't work for me."

"Whatever happened to Trent or Jack or whatever his name was?"
"Jake. He went to a different college after high school. We weren't really together. He just took me to the Prom." At the mention of the word, her face flushed scarlet. She hadn't meant to bring it up.

He rested his chin on his arms. She had seen him do that many times before when he had come to her room to talk. She'd forgotten how much she missed that.
"You know...I'm not that person anymore."
She nodded. "I know."
"No, I don't think you do."

Lois didn't like where the conversation was headed. She changed the subject.
"So you're really going to Mabel's party?"
"For a little bit."

"It's going to be a bunch of teenage girls."
"Are you worried about me? Or them?"
"No, I... I just thought it would be boring for you," Lois said, flustered. "Wouldn't you like to do something else?"

"Are you going to the party?"

"No, I'm just going to help set up. Then I'll give Mabel her birthday present and go."

"Go where?"
"My room."
He chuckled. "Your room? That's not too exciting. Why don't you come with me?"
"Where?"

"I'll take you into town. There's a place I'd like to show you."
"Ok."

He rose out of the chair.
"Seamus?"
He looked over at her.
"I really am glad you're back."
He gave her a soft smile then left the room.

With a sigh of relief, Lois threw the comforter off. She rose off of the bed and stripped out of her underwear, especially her panties.
They were a little too wet.

**Chapter 2**

The next day was Friday. The temperatures were forecast to reach into the upper nineties, so Lois decided to repeat her activities from the previous day. She would invite her friend, Rita, over and they would swim off the family dock.

Her mother was in the kitchen when Lois came down for breakfast. Cathy was a lovely woman and the source of her daughters' good looks. Soft spoken, she was not quick to anger like her husband.  Rather, her temper was a slow burn. She allowed a person just enough rope to hang themselves.

Lois and Mabel's father, Brian, had been one of the casualties of the Gulf War and the girls had never really known him. Cathy had received help from the grandparents on both sides, but she had been the one who had really raised the girls. The three were very close.

"Remember, you've got to come home by three today," Cathy said. "I need help with some of the preparations for the party."
"Will the air conditioning be fixed by then?"
"It should be. Tim said they'd be here around noon."
"Where's Mabel going to be? Is she helping out?"
"Mabel's gone out with Seamus for the day."

Lois was pouring a glass of orange juice and almost spilled the whole thing. She had to set the jug down before juice sloshed all over the hardwood floor.
"She's with Seamus?"

"She said she needed to do some shopping and he offered to take her into town."
"Mom, do you think that's wise?"

Cathy had been composing a shopping list for the party. She looked up at her daughter, eyes peering over the top of her glasses.

"Why not?"

"Well..." Lois said, struggling to come up with a plausible answer.

"Seamus is a responsible man. I'm sure he'll keep Mabel in line."

Lois bit her lip. A question stood on the tip of her tongue; she was almost afraid to ask.

"Mom, did you buy Mabel a baby-doll nightie with matching G-string?"

Her mother nodded. "Yes. She asked me for it."

"But, she's only seventeen."

Cathy set her pen down. "I know it's unconventional, but it's what she asked for.  Besides, she is going to be eighteen."

"But you don't wear that kind of nightie unless you want someone to see it," Lois protested.

"I was eighteen when I bought my first nightie," her mother said, "and mine was worse than the one Mabel chose. At least I helped her pick something suitable."

"You helped her pick it out?" Lois was horrified.

"Lois, isn't this your sister's business?" Cathy said, turning back to the list. "When you were eighteen, you asked for a car."

Yeah, but I wasn't planning to have sex in it, Lois thought to herself. Suddenly a memory, laced with guilt, assaulted her senses. Though she hadn't planned it, she had lost her virginity in that car. The thought silenced her.

Cathy looked up at her again, a sad smile tugging at her lips. "I know it's hard, Baby. You've been looking after Mabel most of her life and now, she's all grown up. You have to let her go and allow her to make her own mistakes. Believe me, this is a lot harder for me than it is for you."

Lois leaned forward to give her mother a hug. She was right. But letting Mabel grow up was part of the problem. She didn't want to think about the other part. Thinking of that hair, that body and those eyes would send her back to her room. And she had no intention of changing her underwear again.
***


Rita arrived later that morning when the heat really began to swelter. Lois had known her ever since she had quit college and joined her family in Hunt's Point. She was a sweet girl and they had met while working in Cathy's little antique shop. The shop had been a present from Tim. He had given it to Cathy when she had announced her need for a hobby.

Rita was not from the wealthier suburbs of Seattle. She was from the city itself, and her attitude was entirely plebeian. Lois felt at home in her company. She was also her one and only confidant.

"I've never met your step-brother, Lo," Rita said as she spread her beach towel out near the dock. The towel was rather thread-bare and Lois laughed to herself about what the neighbors would say if they could get close enough to see it.

"But I feel like I know him, the way you've talked about him. If I had to sum him up in two words, I'd say he's a bad boy."

Lois had just finished applying her sunblock. She was laying back to accept the rays of the sun on her tan skin. Her blue bikini was modest by today's standards. "Oh, he's that all right. Mabel says she thinks he just got out of prison, but I don't think so. He did a lot of wild things as a kid, but never anything criminal." She adjusted her sunglasses.

"Hey you two!" A voice suddenly called.
"OMG!" Rita said, rising up on her elbow and peering over her shades. "Speak of the devil..."

Lois looked up in alarm. Mabel walked toward them with Seamus in tow. Both were dressed for swimming, though Mabel's suit left little to the imagination. Lois hoped that she wouldn't bend over and pop the

Brazilian-cut bottom off.

Seamus wore sunglasses, so she had no idea where his eyes were looking. She wondered if he was admiring her curves.
"Hey, Mabel! Nice bikini." Rita said.
"Thanks! I just got it. Had to try on hundreds of them before I could find this one. It's an original Dortini."

"Ugh," Lois said under her breath.
"Never heard of him," Rita said.
"He's up and coming," Mabel replied. "At least, that's what the saleslady said. By the way, I don't think you've met Seamus."

"No, I haven't. Nice to meet you."
Seamus nodded. He'd always been rather shy around strangers. It didn't seem like three years had changed that very much.

"Lo talks about you all the time."
Lois shot her one time confidant a look. The girl had suddenly forgotten how to keep a secret.
"All good I hope," he said. He lowered the shades.
"She says you're a bad boy."

Lois cringed. She wanted nothing more, at that moment, then to jump into the lake and sink.
"She did?" Seamus raised his eyebrows.
"It's ok. Most girls like bad boys."
"C'mon, Rita!" Lois said, jumping to her feet.

"What?"

"We're going swimming."

"But—"

Lois grabbed her arm and dragged her toward the lake.

"What are you doing!" she exclaimed once they were in the water and out of earshot. "I told you that stuff in confidence! You're not supposed to tell anyone, especially him!"

"Geez, Lo, calm down."

"I will not! I didn't want him to know I thought of him that way."

"He's your step-brother. Why would he care what you think?"

"That's beside the point. I just didn't want him to know."

"Oh my gosh," Rita said in a hushed voice. "You have the hots for him!"

"Stop being ridiculous," Lois huffed.

"You do!"

"That's sick, Rita."

"He's not related to you. What's sick about it?" she looked back toward Seamus and Mabel. They were swimming a few yards off. "Obviously, Mabel doesn't think it's sick."

"Mabel has questionable taste."

"Really? I don't think she does."

"Let's talk about something else," Lois grumbled. "I don't want to talk about this anymore. And you shouldn't either—to anybody!"

"Alright already," Rita grinned. "You're such a grouch--I think you need to get laid."

Lois had overcome her embarrassment, but she still didn't really want to talk to Seamus or Mabel. After dinner, Rita went home and Lois went to her room. She spent the rest of the evening listening to music. Now that the air conditioning had been fixed, it was much more comfortable in her room. She still kept the window open however, just to hear the sounds of the lake.

In between songs, Lois heard a whistling coming from outside. She rose off of her bed went to the window. In the purple twilight, Seamus walked below. He whistled the tune of the song she had just played. At the precise moment that she looked down, he looked up. The tune faded on his lips. They stared at one another; then he winked.

She hadn't meant to smile, but she did. Afraid that her expression was a little too warm, too inviting, she ducked back into her room before he could take it the wrong way.

## Chapter 3

Saturday morning went by quickly. Lois had so much

to do, what with decorating and helping her mother make the birthday dinner. Cathy liked to cook as much as she liked antiques and, as a result, Tim didn't employ a cook. In fact, servants were few and far between in the O'Reilly household.

The guests began to arrive just before dinner. Most of them were friends who had graduated with Mabel. There would be twenty-five girls in all.

Before the house became too inundated with loud, giggly rich girls, Lois pulled her sister into her bedroom and  gave her her present. Mabel unwrapped it with gusto.

"Oh, Lois! It's beautiful!" Mabel cried, holding up the little snow globe. Within the glass orb, a carousel pony pranced. Mabel shook it and the pony was obscured by a storm of glitter. "You got the one I liked! Thank you!"
"You're welcome, Sissy," Lois said, using her sister's pet name. "Happy Birthday!"

Mabel jumped up to hug her sister. "Oh, I've got to show the girls. I love it!" She hurried out of the room. Lois was cleaning up the wrapping paper when a knock came on the door. She opened it to find Seamus standing in the hallway.  He wore a black t-shirt and jeans. She hadn't realized before how much he had grown. He seemed to tower over her now. "Ready to go?" he asked.

"Oh, I don't know if I should go now," she said. "They haven't had dinner yet."

"I'm going to buy us some," he said.

"Oh, well...alright."

"I already told your mom we were going so we can just sneak out. Come on."

"But I'm not dressed," she said. "Shorts and a tank top aren't proper dinner attire."

"Where we're going it doesn't matter." He held out his hand to her.

She took it and he led her toward the rear of the house. They hurried out the back door and into the early evening.

Seamus's car, a 1996 Cobra Mystic, was parked in the garage. In certain light and at certain angles, the color of the paint seemed to shift and flow. The base coat was green, but purple, gold and amber could emerge at any given moment.

When she slipped into the car, the smell of leather seats and Seamus's aftershave wafted over her. She inhaled deeply.

"What is your aftershave called?" she asked.

"I don't wear aftershave. Just deodorant."

"Oh."

He started the car and pulled out of the garage.

They talked a little as he drove. She was too uncomfortable to ask where he had been for the last three years, so she kept the conversation light.

The area he took her to was unfamiliar. It seemed to be the seedier side of Seattle, a place she had never been, nor did she want to go. He drove down several side streets until they reached a building with a large neon sign.

The sign was the cartoon representation of a woman wearing a red dress. She was bent over, exposing her rear. The sign read: TURN THE OTHER CHEEK. According to the sign, alcohol was not allowed in the building.

It was a full-nude strip club.

Lois's scowled as they parked on the side of the brick building. She turned to Seamus, ready to spit venom. "What is this? A strip club? What makes you think I'm the kind of girl who wants to go there?"

"I don't think you're the kind of girl who would go there."

"Then why are we here?"

"Because we're going in there." He pointed to the storefront next door.

The simple sign hanging in front read: JIM'S GYM.

"A gym?"

"Yeah. Of course, if you'd like to go to the strip club..."

"No, no, that's ok." Lois's cheeks were burning now.

She jumped out of the car.

The gym was well-lit and clean smelling. One area housed various exercise machines, while the other area seemed to be entirely devoted to the sport of boxing. Speed bags and heavy bags lined the wall while the center of the room was dominated by a regulation boxing ring. Two men in headgear were sparring in the middle of it.

An elderly man dressed in a grey hoodie and sweat pants watched the sparring match. He shouted out advice as the two men fought.

"That guy is the father of one of my friends. He used to be a great manager back in the day."
"He looks like Burgess Meredith," Lois observed.
The elderly man caught sight of Seamus and beckoned him over. They joined him at the apron of the ring.
"What's up, Irish?" he asked.
"Nothin' much. Is Al here?"

"Nope. He'll be here around six, though, if you want to wait around." He favored Lois with a cursory glance. "She from next door?"

"Yeah, her name is Roxy."
"It is not!" Lois cried. She held out a hand. "I'm Lois Carmody."
"Nick Spinetti." He turned to Seamus. "Women sap your strength, Irish."

Seamus smiled. "Thanks for the warning, Nick."

He gave Lois a quick tour. She burned with curiosity and when they had stopped by one of the available speed bags, she asked, "What do you do here?"

"I work out." He began to punch the speed bag.

"Are you a boxer?"

"It's just a hobby. I've been in a few fights. Nothing spectacular."

"How long have you been doing this?"

"About two years."

The bag was really moving now.

"Well, if it ain't the mick," a man called out. He was big, much larger than Seamus. The fluorescent lights lent a shine to his bald head.

Seamus grabbed the bag and halted its progress. His eyes were focused straight ahead, his mouth forming a grim line.

"What are you doing on my bag, mick?" the big man said. "You finally gonna train for our match?"

"Let's go," he said to Lois, taking her hand.

"Hidin' behind a woman, mick?" the man called after them. "You pussy!"

Seamus led Lois over to Nick. "Tell Al I'll see him next time, would ya, Nick?"

The old man nodded. "It ain't none of my business, Irish, but someday..."

"I know, I'll have to knock him on his ass. Just...not today."

The old man shrugged.
The bald man was still calling after them, when they walked out the door.

## Chapter 4

"Sorry about that," he said as they drove away.
"It's no problem," Lois said. "Is that guy always like that?"
"Yeah. We've never gotten along."
"What's wrong with him?"
"He's a dick."
Lois giggled.

"Who's this Al you went in to see?"
"My buddy. Nick's kid. He's the one who got me into boxing. Ok, here we are."
Seamus pulled into a drive-thru sandwich place and quickly ordered their dinner. He drove back to Tim and Cathy's home.

"Are we going back already?" Lois asked, disappointed.
"No, we're not going to the party. We're going down to the lake."
"We are?"

"Don't worry, you won't need your suit."

The words "skinny dipping" suddenly leaped to Lois's mind. She imagined them both naked in the water while twenty-six teenage girls giggled at them.

But, Seamus had no interest in swimming at all. He took her to a more isolated part of the property and together, they ate the sandwiches he had bought.
"I have missed talking to you, Lois," Seamus gazed out over the lake. The sun had dropped low in the sky, taking some of the heat with it.
"I've missed out conversations too. You always had something interesting to tell me or funny to say. It got boring after you left."

Seamus wadded up one of the paper wrappers that had covered his sandwich and tossed it aside. "I ran into someone today," he said.
"Oh? I didn't know you'd gone out."

"It was your friend Rita."
Lois immediately put up her guard. "What did she have to say?"
"Not too much. We talked about her work, stuff like that."

"That's good." Relief crept in. Rita had finally learned to keep her mouth shut.
"She did say one interesting thing, though."
Lois put her sandwich aside. It suddenly tasted sour and the texture seemed mealy. "What was that?"
"It had to do with you."

"Really?" she felt the flush spreading over her skin.
"Yeah, she said you had the hots for me."
Lois laughed. The sound was a trifle too loud and a bit too hysterical.
"That silly girl!"

He watched her carefully, his lips untouched by a smile. Desire burned in his eyes. It was unmistakable. She suddenly became aware of where she was. The place was lonely and far enough from the house that no one would hear her should she cry out.

"Rita was making that up," Lois tried to sound convincing, but the tremor in her voice betrayed her.
"Was she?" His eyes scorched her. He reached out to take hold of her wrist. She wanted to snatch it away, but for some reason her arm wouldn't obey. He placed his fingers on her pulse.
"Sure is moving fast."
His grip on her intensified. She realized, too late, that she was trapped.

Panic flickered in her eyes. She knew he saw it.
"Just answer two questions and I'll let you go," His tone was slow, measured. It was as though he were talking to a frightened deer instead of her.
"A-Alright."

"Do you think it would be disgusting to be with me?"
The word came quickly and unbidden. She was

terrified when she heard it.
"No."

His grip relaxed.
The next question he asked was more difficult. "Then why can't we be together?"

She didn't have a ready answer for this one.
She wanted to say it was because he was her step-brother, but she knew that was a lie.
When she didn't answer, he answered for her.
"It's because of Prom, isn't it?"

She looked up at him. The nod was almost imperceptible.
He released her.
Lois rose to her feet. She just wanted to get away now.

He stared out over the lake. "People change," he said as she was beginning to leave. "And sometimes, the person they were before still haunts them."
Lois wanted to answer, but the pain in her stomach and the accompanying nausea wouldn't allow it. She hurried away.

## Chapter 5

Lois avoided Seamus for a few days, too confused to face him. By the time she had come to an understanding of herself, she realized that the avoidance appeared to be mutual. Seamus had moved on.

Mabel had been angry with her for leaving with Seamus during the party, but soon forgot everything when he began to spend more time with her. They were together nearly every day. Tim and Cathy seemed oblivious of what was happening between them, but Lois wasn't.

The events of that Saturday night and Seamus's change toward her, depressed her. She started feeling strange. It was almost as though she were sick. She had no real symptoms, just a general malaise, but it seemed like something more than that. She couldn't figure it out.

Tim and Cathy had planned a day just for the family in order to celebrate Mabel's birthday in their own private way. They were all supposed to have dinner at Tango, followed by a show at the Paramount Theater. Lois begged off, saying that she felt too ill to go. She wasn't up to being ignored by Seamus. When they had left, she went back to bed.

Lois awoke later that afternoon, sweating. She rose and checked the thermostat in her room. The temperature was too high and no cool air came from the vent. The air conditioner must have broken down again. She sighed. Nothing seemed to be going right in this house lately.

Thinking that she might be experiencing a little heat exhaustion, she decided to take a shower. The thought of cool water streaming over her body was very appealing.

Mabel, Seamus and Lois shared the only bathroom on the second floor. Tim had talked about adding another bathroom, but hadn't gotten around to it as yet. Lois couldn't wait until he did. She was tired of waiting for Mabel in the mornings.

Since no one was home, she didn't bother to close the door nor did she bring her clothes in. She would simply do what she always did when no one was home--undress in her room, run in and take her shower, then run back to her room. It saved time and she didn't have to clean up the bathroom up afterward.

She was already in the bathroom, ready to step into the shower, when she noticed the lack of soap. "Damn it, Mabel," she grumbled as she hurried to the hall closet. "You're supposed to keep this stocked." The soap on the top shelf was almost out of her reach. She had to jump to get it.

When she returned to the bathroom, the shower was running. Lois stood before the drawn shower curtain, puzzled. She didn't remember turning it on.
The heat must be making her forgetful. With a shrug, she pulled the curtain back.

A light spray hit her face and misted over her body.
Though the water was tepid, it felt like ice.
Seamus stood in the stall, staring at her.

## Chapter 6

Lois stayed rooted to the spot, clutching the curtain.
Her heart pounded with a thunderous roar.
Rivulets of water rushed over his torso, arm and legs.
She tracked one as it sped down over his abdomen
and into the thatch of dark hair below his waist.

Against her will, she focused on what lay beyond.
His member grew erect before her, as though it were
saluting. It seemed much larger than last time.
Her pulse quickened even more and a warm flush rose
in her body.

Seamus seemed to recover more quickly than she. He
reached out, grasped her about the waist and pulled
her into the stall. The box of soap slipped from her
fingers and hit the floor with a soft thud.

She threw her arms around his neck and met his lips
hungrily, allowing him to pull her tightly against him.
Every inch of him was cool and wet.

His tongue delved into her mouth as his left hand
roved over the curve of her hip. Then the fingers of his
right hand traced their way down to her mound and

inside her cleft. When he touched the fold of flesh that formed her clitoris, she felt a jolt of electricity go through her body. He released her from the kiss.
His touch was like fire and the flames licked at her, spreading from her loins into every part of her body. Despite the heat, she shivered.

With one hand, he clutched the small of her back as the fingers of the other gently massaged the source of her pleasure. She moaned, clutching his shoulder. Seamus turned and pinned her against the wall. His height had shielded her from the water before, but now it gushed over her. At the same time, he inserted a finger within the secret center of her body. She gasped, her eyes snapping open.

Lois watched his face as he pleasured her. His desire was obvious and it seemed to spike higher every time she cried out. He continued on until the orgasm rose over her. She dug her fingernails into his shoulders as she leaned against him. Tiny half-moons the color of blood, appeared on his skin.

"I want you!" she panted. "Oh, now...please!"
He moved to enter her but the disparity in their heights wouldn't allow for it.
"Turn around," he said hoarsely, guiding her body so that she now faced the wall. He tried to enter, but was once again denied.

Desperation seemed to replace desire in his eyes. He

threw the curtain open, and stepped out of the shower, beckoning her to join him.

She stepped on the edge and he lifted her into his arms. He carried her out of the bathroom and toward his own room.

The door was half-closed. He kicked it open with one foot and rushed in taking her to the bed.

Her ardor had not cooled during the journey from bath to bedroom, but instead increased. She pulled him on top of her, arching her back and raising her hips to allow him easy admission. He slid into her, and she raised her knees so that she might squeeze his hips.

Three years ago, she had wondered what he would feel like inside. As the silken head, and shaft entered fully, her question was finally answered.

His lips found her throat and the intensity of the pleasure he gave her suddenly increased ten-fold. She cried out, trying to push him back, but he remained where he was. His pace increased bringing another plateau of pleasure upon her. It crushed her, leaving her gasping for breath.

When it had passed, she rose renewed. His rhythm became deep and quick. She matched it with her hips, allowing deeper access as she did. Another orgasm rushed through her like a tsunami. As she rode it out, he suddenly groaned, his eyes widening. He pulled away from her, panting as he fought to gain control. Water dripped from his hair, onto her stomach. The climax was still raw within her, and each droplet afforded her another shiver of pleasure.

"We've got to get a condom," he announced. "I almost lost it there."

She rose up on her elbows. "Do you have any?"
He shook his head.
"Do you... take birth control?"
"No."

"What about Dad and Cathy?"
"I doubt it. Mom went into menopause last summer." He glanced at the door. She followed his eyes then answered his unvoiced question.
"No, Mabel doesn't. She doesn't use birth control either. I looked."
"You looked?"
"I worry about her, especially..."
"Since I came back?"
"Well..."

He shook his head. "Don't you know by now, I only see her as a sister. And a little sister at that. There's a huge difference between you two."
Lois grinned.
He looked down at his still swollen member.

"Well, look at this for instance. I haven't even lost my erection. If that's not love, I don't know what is." His

face suddenly flushed red and he averted his eyes.
A little pain, dull and sweet, touched her heart.
When he turned back to face her, she held her arms out to him. "We don't need one. You can just pull out."

His lips formed that strange, grim line once more, and he shook his head.
"No," he said softly. "Not that way."
He pulled her up into his arms and held her, a shudder wracking his body.
"Why?"

"Can't do that to you."
She reached down and placed a tentative hand about his penis. The minute she touched it, a soft moan escaped his lips.
"Has it been a while?" she asked.
"Three years," he replied.
Lois raised her eyebrows. "Wow!"

She began to stroke him, alternating the amount of pressure as she did so.
He gripped her wrist and gently pushed her back. She waited a few moments, watching him as he held her at arm's length. Then she pushed forward and kissed him. He fell back with her on top of him.

Before he could stop her, she moved to take his penis into her mouth. He moaned as she began to stroke the shaft, her tongue swirling about the head in a counter-clockwise motion. He bucked against her but she didn't falter.

He tasted sweet when he finished.

## Chapter 7

Lois lay in his arms afterward. There was a dull ache in her heart, making it difficult for her to breathe.
She studied the nipple of the naked man. There was something wrong about it. She reached out, brushing her finger against it. It felt wrong. When she touched it again, she realized that it was scar tissue.
"This is a bullet wound," she exclaimed.

He lay silent, watching her as she turned his arm over to investigate the other side. There was an eagle tattooed there. Its dark eye was an exit wound.
"What happened?"
"Firefight. In Afghanistan."
"You were in the army?"
"For two years,"

Tears welled up within her. She tried to stave them off, but one escaped and trickled down her cheek.
"It's alright," he said. "I'm alright...now."
"How did it happen?"
He sighed. "They were in the wrong place at the wrong time. Or maybe we were. I forget." He pulled his arm away, examined it and then dropped it by his side.

"I met Al in the army."
Lois didn't press him on the subject. Instead, she flowed with him.

"Is that where you got into boxing?"
He nodded. "I was messed up." He looked at her and grinned. "Well, you already knew that. Anyway, I met Al in a bar fight. We got out before the M.P.s arrived and became friends. He said that I was a loose cannon and it would get me killed someday. So he introduced me to boxing. When we got back last year, I came up here to train under his dad."

 "That day we went to the gym, and that bald guy started taunting you, it's the first time I ever saw you refuse a fight. I knew you weren't scared of him."
"No, I'm not scared of him. I'm scared of me."
Seamus replied.
***
Lois was filled with a sweet melancholy when she returned to her room to dress. They had slipped into a different world for a few hours, and she wasn't anxious to return.

She was slipping into her blouse when he came to her room. He leaned against the door jamb, his hands in the pockets of his jeans.

"I don't think we should tell anyone...yet," she said.
He nodded, his eyes on the floor.

"It's not that I don't want them to know, it's just—it's complicated."

"Yeah."

She came to him and he wrapped his arms around her.

"I suppose you're right. I don't know what Dad will think," he said.

"I don't think Mom would mind. She's pretty liberal about everything. But, Mabel... Mabel won't understand."

"She'll get over it."

"I don't know. Let's just keep it quiet for a while."

"Alright." He began to bend toward her, lips parted. The front door slammed.

"Lois! Lois don't tell me you're in bed!" Mabel called up the stairs.

He kissed her gently. Then returned to his room. Lois hurried down the stairs.

"I'm awake. Did you have fun?"

"I did! The show was awesome! Did Seamus get back yet?"

"I think he's in his room."

"I was so bummed when he said he had some chores to do today. I can't wait to tell him about the show." She rushed up the stairs.

Her mother and Tim entered the foyer.

"Oh no. Did the air conditioner break again?" he

asked.

"Feels like it." Lois replied.
"Damn. They told me it would be fixed this time."
"Are you feeling better, Lois?" her mother asked.
Mabel descended the stairs with Seamus. Lois glanced up at him, then back at her mother.
"I'm fine now," she said.

## Chapter 8

When Lois awoke the next morning, Seamus had gone. Her mother told her that he had gone into town and didn't know when he'd be back.

She waited most of the day for his return. He finally came home, close to three in the afternoon. She watched him park his car in the garage but instead of going directly to the house, he joined his father out back. Tim stood over the repairman who was trying to fix the air conditioning system. She went out to them
"So you got your own place?" she heard Tim say.
She stopped, still out of view.

"Yeah, I'll be moving in tomorrow."
"Good. Coming to work on Thursday?"
"Yup."
"You know, you don't have to start at the bottom. You're my son."

"Which is why I want to work my way up."

Tim reached into his back pocket and pulled out his wallet. "Take this," he said pulling out several hundred dollar bills.

"I can't take that, Dad."
"You can and you will. It's an advance, not a handout. You're going to need money for furniture, if nothing else."

Neither of them appeared to have seen her, so she turned around and walked back inside. Seamus was leaving. Her heart felt heavy as it throbbed in her breast. Tears blurred her vision. She took a deep breath and turned toward the kitchen.
Cathy sat at the table, perusing a cookbook.
"I think I'll go back to work early, Mom," she announced.

"But, you've got three more days off," her mother replied. "Rita can handle things until you get back." Just then, Seamus walked in. He walked past Lois without a word and greeted Cathy.

"Got some news for you," he announced. "I've got my own apartment. I'm moving out tomorrow."
"Oh," Cathy said, sounding disappointed. "We were hoping you'd stay a little longer. It's been so nice having you back with us."

He cast a sideways glance at Lois. "I'm sorry. I just can't stay here any longer. I'm used to being on my own."

Lois stormed out of the room. She heard his footsteps behind her as she rushed out the front door.
"Where are you going?" he called after her.
She turned, and pointed a finger at him. Her voice was quiet, yet harsh. "I am not a one night stand!"
Before he could say another word, she rushed for her car.

"Lois! Lois, come back here!"
She jammed the key into the ignition and backed out of the driveway at an almost reckless speed.
She didn't go to the antique store. Instead, she drove around aimlessly for hours before returning home. When she arrived, she went straight up to her room. Her pillow was soaked by the time she fell asleep.
***

Sometime after midnight, she awoke to the gentle creak of her door as it opened. A shadow slipped in and as it approached, she rose to her elbow. She reached toward the lamp and with a swift twist, light flooded the room.

"What are you doing here?" she asked coldly.
"I'm here to talk to you," Seamus said, "and you're going to listen."
"Am I?"
"I do not think you are a one night stand."
"Then why are you leaving?"
He sat at the edge of her bed.

"A friend of mine offered me the place a week ago, but I wasn't sure I wanted it until yesterday."

"You still haven't answered my question."

"I wanted a place where we can have privacy. I don't want to..." he paused. "...to make love to you here. I don't want it to be quick or sneaky. I don't want to worry about somebody walking in."

The color drained from Lois's face and she buried it in her hands.

"Don't cry."

"Oh, I'm not. I'm just...oh, please don't look at me!"

He tried to pull her hands away, but she hid in the blanket.

He lifted her chin. Her face was burned with a furious blush.

"I've managed to humiliate myself—again!" she wailed.

He grinned. "You're still pretty though."

Her blush increased and he kissed her.

"I am so sorry," she said.

"I keep trying to tell you I've changed."

"I know."

"Yesterday, before you ran away, I was going to take you over there and show you the place. Would you like to go tomorrow?"

"Sure."

"Good." He rose to go.

"You're going?" she said softly.

He didn't look at her. 'Lois, I can barely keep my hands off you as it is. I think my leaving is a good idea right now." He walked toward the door.

"Goodnight." she called after him.

"Goodnight."

As he turned toward his room, his shadow in the hall revealed the effect she had had on him. Lois hid her face in the damp pillow and squealed.

**Chapter 9**

Seamus's new apartment was in a middle class suburb of Seattle. The building was tall, distinguished and made of red brick. His apartment was on the sixth-floor corner and afforded a breathtaking view of the city.

Lois walked across the hardwood floors and gazed out the large picture windows. "It's beautiful," she said. "The bedroom is over here," he said, directing her down the hall. She followed him into the spacious room. A laugh escaped her lips when she saw what occupied it.

"When did you get that?" she asked.

Seamus flopped on the bed. "It was delivered this morning. But, wait!" He rose and hurried to the closet.

Lois surveyed the bare room. There were blinds on the windows and a hook in the beam which ran across the ceiling, but little else.

"What's that for?" She pointed  at the hook when Seamus emerged from the closet.

"The hook is for this."

He handed her an item packaged in plastic. It was a strange contraption, with various bits of hardware and Velcro straps. Some of it was black and some was leopard print. The cardboard picture within the packaging depicted a half-naked woman suspended from the ceiling, her feet and hands strapped. She appeared to be seated in a swing.

"Oh...my...gosh!" she said. "You're into bondage?"

Seamus pulled a notebook from his back pocket. He wrote in it and then tore the page out before handing it to Lois. The word ASSUME, was printed on it. He had circled "Ass".

"When you assume..." he prompted.

"You make an ass out of you and me," she finished. "Although this device can be used that, it isn't why I got it."

"Oops." she smiled sheepishly.

"By the way," he said holding up a small cellophane wrapped square. "This time, I've come prepared."

Once the swing was suspended from the hook, he turned to her.

"Come here."

She moved into his arms and he began to undress her. He removed her tank top and bra, then he pushed her backward onto the bed. Her flip-flops and shorts came next, and finally her panties. He pulled them off slowly, sliding them along her legs and before tossing them on the floor.

He undressed while she watched. Then he moved toward her.

She spread her legs in anticipation, thinking he would soon be on top of her. Instead, Seamus held his hands out to help her up. He lifted her into his arms, carried her to the swing, and strapped her in.

She stood in the device and looked into his eyes. The swing had solved the problem of height disparity. Seamus stepped up to her and she spread her legs so that she could wrap them around his waist. He licked a finger and winked at her before lowering it to stroke her. He rubbed her lightly until she became slick inside.

Her body tensed against him and she bit her lip as he entered. The swing allowed him to penetrate more deeply and as he held her against him, her breathing came in ragged gasps. He slowly pistoned in and out, and she leaned back, eyes closed, lips curled in an ecstatic smile.

He leaned over and took her right nipple between his lips, teasing the outer edge with his tongue. She felt the orgasm rising within her, bursting through her body, and she cried out. His name was on her lips and the word seemed to stimulate him, for his pace increased every time she spoke it.

She rose and this time, leaned forward to wrap her arms around his neck. His hands ran through her hair, raising a delicious chill along the outside of her skin. He continued to pump into her as she squeezed his hips with her thighs.

His body rubbed against that tender, tiny part of her. Pleasure joined pleasure and she cried out as another climax surged through her body. The tips of her fingers and those of her toes tingled.

He didn't stop. Instead, he increased his pace. Her grip on him tightened until he suddenly pulled away.
He picked up the condom, pulled it from its plastic wrapper, and quickly sheathed his member. The action was fluid and took only a matter of seconds. He didn't seem to skip a beat.
She shivered at his touch. It was like embracing a pleasant electric shock.

Seamus groaned. It was a deeply masculine sound and it triggered another climax within her. She cried out as he grasped her tightly, his body spasming in release. He held her, kissing her throat and earlobes as she panted, clutching him. Red furrows, caused by her nails covered the skin of his left shoulder. He released her from the swing and returned with her to the bed. They lay side by side, staring at the ceiling.

"Can I ask you something?" she said. The afternoon sun had by now made its tour of the room. It stood in the western sky, shining through the glass, casting a golden glow over their bodies and onto the bed.
"Go ahead."

"What in the world did you and Tim fight over that night?"
He stared at the ceiling so long, she thought he wasn't going to answer.
"Denise," he said at last.
"Denise Allen? Your Prom date?"

He nodded. "She claimed I got her pregnant and wanted Dad to pay her off. He told me I had to do right by her and take responsibility for the baby. I told him that she was lying, but he didn't believe me. He never believed me back then."

"Was that because of what happened with your mom in Anaheim?"
He turned sharply, his eyes searching hers. "You know about that?"
"I overheard some things. I don't know everything."
"You know about Louie?"
She shook her head.

"He's the guy my mom left my dad for. Real piece of crap. She used to leave me with him when she went out during the day. When she was gone, he'd beat me. He'd never hit me in the face, or hard enough to put me in the hospital, but he'd do enough to hurt. I remember. He used to cuff my ear. God, I hated that."

"My mom always sided with him. He'd say I fell downplaying, or he had to discipline me. When I started calling Dad about it, they got scared. Mom would cry, ask why I was lying, why I didn't want to be with her. He'd threaten me that it would be worse next time. So, when Dad came, I wouldn't say anything." He swallowed. "I was too scared."

"Tim stopped believing you?"

He nodded. "The last time I called, Louie had beaten me worse than usual. He gave me a black eye and I finally had proof. I called Dad, but he didn't come. When that happened, they knew Dad wouldn't be a problem. They weren't scared anymore."

"What did you do?" she asked softly. Her lower lip trembled.

"I realized that I couldn't be scared anymore because if I was, he'd kill me. Nobody could protect me, so I protected myself. The next time she left me with him, I had a baseball bat. I sent him to the hospital. After that, she let me go. She didn't want me back."

"Did you tell your Dad?"

"My mom told him what I had done and he paid them

to keep it quiet. He believed her. Never asked for my version."

"Oh, Seamus..." Her voice was choked with tears. He pulled her close. "Don't feel sorry for me," he said softly. "It took a while and I had to overcome a lot of bitterness, but I worked hard to own this. I'm no victim. I even forgave Dad."

"I wish it had never happened to you."
"I wouldn't be who I am if it hadn't. I'll tell you one thing for damn sure. I won't allow it to happen to anyone else."

She hugged him fiercely.
"Enough about me. Tell me what you've been up to these three years. Tell me why you left college."
"It's stupid,"

"Tell me."
"There was a guy after Jake. We were serious for a while. I thought we'd get married."
"He had different ideas?"

She shook her head.
"You had different ideas?"
"I found out I didn't love him. I loved somebody else."
"And that guy, the somebody else, what happened with him?"

"He left before he knew I loved him. I waited for him,

but I was scared when he came back. I'm not scared anymore." She stared into his eyes.

He squeezed her and kissed her lips.
"It's kinda funny. You know I haven't slept with anyone in the last three years. You are the first since the night you caught me with Denise."
"I thought that was strange. I thought you'd have slept with tons of women by now."

"I didn't want tons of women. That night, and every night after, I just wanted you. I guess, even then, I loved you."

She would have rolled on top of him and started their love making all over again, if the knock hadn't come on the door. He looked at her, puzzled.
"I didn't give anybody but you and Al this address," he said. "And Al could've called."

He rose. The knocking became insistent.
"I'm coming, I'm coming!" he said, throwing on his jeans. He hurried out of the room.
Lois didn't recognize the voice of the person at the door. She rose and dressed, straining to hear the conversation but not able to make out what they were saying. She walked down the hall and entered the living room. A tall black man stood just inside the door. He introduced himself as Al Spinetti.

"So this is your friend, Al." Lois held out a hand for her

to shake.

"And you must be Lois. I've heard a great deal about you. Seems like all he talked about for three whole years was you."

"As you can see, Rita and Al would get along great," Seamus said. "But you still haven't told me the reason for this visit. What is this matter of life and death that can't be explained over the phone?"

"Luke Morgan was in a car accident last night. He'll be ok, but going to be in the hospital for a while."

"Damn." Seamus ran his hands through his hair. "He was supposed to fight Lead Head in three months. What's your dad going to do about it?"

"He told me to come and get you, Irish. I'm not allowed to come home without you."

"Who is Lead Head?" Lois asked.

"He's the dick with the bald head," Seamus said. "I won't fight that guy."

"Now's not the time to play the Quiet Man, Irish. Dad really needs you. He's sunk a lot of money into this fight. In fact, he was going to sign Lead Head in the morning. But, after this, it's likely he'll drop out. The only person he wants more than Morgan is you."

Seamus stared at the floor, his lips pulled tight. Then he sighed. "Alright, I'll come with you."

"Good" Al smiled.

"Can I come too?" Lois asked.

"Sure. Come for dinner if you'd like."

"Let me finish getting dressed and we'll get going."

Seamus ducked into the bedroom.

"So I hear I've got you to thank for getting Seamus on track and into boxing. I guess you kind of saved his life," she said.

"Saved his life?" the big man shook his head. "No, I didn't save his life. He saved mine."

Lois wanted to ask what he meant by that, but Seamus came back out, now fully dressed.

"Let's go." he said, slipping his wallet and keys into the pockets of his jeans.

## Chapter 10

Al's parents lived in an apartment above Jim's Gym. Nick's wife, Cora, a beautiful black woman of fifty or so, met them at the door and led them into the living room.

"Hiya Roxy," Nick said, as they entered the living room. He sat before the TV, a beer in his hand.

"Hello again," Lois said with a smile. The mischievous glint in his eye told her that he knew her real name. The family accepted her immediately, and she felt very much at home. Seamus took her on a tour, while Cora finished preparing the steak dinner and Al sat down to watch television with his father.

The place was neat and well-furnished. It featured a

wall dedicated to the art of pugilism, filled with photos of the boxers Nick had trained over the years.

Lois searched the wall for a picture of Seamus. She found one in the corner and read the date. The picture had been taken the previous year.
Seamus pointed out some of the people he knew personally. He was quite animated as talked about the different boxers and Lois was captivated by his stories.

A framed photo of Al in uniform hung near the bottom of the wall and another that featured Al and Seamus together in fatigues. Lois pointed it out, but Seamus passed over it quickly. He moved to the opposite side of the wall.

Soon, dinner was served.
"There's so much food," Lois whispered, as they sat down to the table. "Did they know we were coming?"
"Nick always eats like this," Seamus whispered back. "You should see what breakfast is like when he has his boxers over."

After the dinner, Lois helped Cora with the dishes. As she carried the dishes into the kitchen, she passed another photo of Al and Seamus. This time, they stood together before what looked like a bleak yet hauntingly beautiful landscape. She paused to examine it.
"That was taken a few days before Irish saved my Al's

life," Cora said.

"What happened?" Lois asked gently.
"Al doesn't talk about it much and he's only given me bits and pieces, but it seems they were attacked one night by a squad of coalition soldiers."
"What? It was friendly fire?"

Cora nodded. "Al's squad was fired upon while walking through a town they thought was clear. It was dark and they were mistaken for the enemy. Al got shot and Irish took a bullet getting him out of there. They were the only ones from their squad who got out alive."

Lois turned back toward the living room. Nick and Al were laughing and Seamus joined in. Her heart suddenly swelled in her breast.
"He's a good man," Cora said.
"Yes," Lois said. "He is."

## Chapter 11

Seamus was quiet after they left Al's parent's place. The night was cool, suggesting that the freakish heat wave had finally ended. They rolled down the car windows instead of using the air conditioning.

"I'm not going to be able to see you like I want to," he said. "What with work and training..."
"I can't come and watch you train?"

"Sorry. Nick says that women make the legs weak. He won't allow it."

She crossed her arms over her chest and sank back into the seat. "He really is Burgess Meredith," she said.

Seamus chuckled.
"Can I come and see you fight?"
"That you can do. The match will be in October. I'd rather you didn't say anything to Dad and Cathy though."

"You don't want them to come?"
"They have an image of me that I'm trying to break. I don't think they'd understand right now. It's going to be hard enough to tell them about you and me."
She nodded.

"I'm going to drop you off at their house and then go home."
"Ok," she said.

He pulled into the driveway thirty minutes later and parked. When he cut the engine, the sounds of night became audible. The trees sighed softly under the influence of a gentle breeze and the crickets sang in reply.

"It's going to be hard to be away from you," she said.
He reached across and took her hand. She squeezed

it. "Can I kiss you?"

He met her as she leaned over, and then kissed her gently on the mouth.

"I can't wait until this is over," she said.
"Me neither," he replied. "Better go in. I'll call you later."

She opened the car door, got out and walked slowly toward the house. He didn't drive away until she reached it. She stood on the porch to watch him go. Cathy was waiting for her in the living room when she entered. Her mother was dressed in a silk robe, her feet tucked beneath her on the couch. She was reading a magazine.

"Hi, Mom," she said.
"Did you eat?" Cathy asked.
"Yes, we got something."
Cathy closed the magazine and peered up at her daughter. A jolt of fear went through Lois's body. She knew that look.

"Is there something you want to tell me?" Cathy asked softly.
Lois's knees were like jelly. She fell into a nearby chair, her mouth dry.
Her mother knew.

"In twenty years you've never been able to hide

anything from me," her mother chided. "You are the most honest person I have ever met. And when you start hiding in your bedroom and avoiding me, I know something's up."

Lois swallowed hard.

"I don't know how to tell you this, Mom" she said, her voice cracking.

"Just do what you always do. Spit it out."

"I'm in love."

"With Seamus?"

A feeling of relaxation flowed through her body as she nodded. It was out.

"Were you worried because he's your step-brother?"

"Kind of."

Her mother clicked her tongue.

"Mostly because of how you and Tim see him. Like he's a bad guy." She rose to her feet. "He's not bad, Mom. He's a good man, a really good man."

"Shh!" her mother cautioned, waving her back into her seat. "You'll wake the whole house."

"Tim's not going to like it. He doesn't understand Seamus. He—"

"Your step-father loves Seamus," Cathy said. "And he loves you. He'll get used to the idea."

"Mabel won't."

"Mabel will...in time."

They were interrupted by a loud crash and the tinkle of broken glass. It came from the second floor.
The two women rushed toward the stairs. When Lois got to the first step, the crunch of glass sounded underfoot. Cathy turned the light on.

Water dripped down the stairs. Glass and glitter were scattered everywhere. A small, carousel pony, broken in two, lay on the third step, next to the cracked base of the snow globe. Lois picked some of the pieces, her fingers sparkling in the amber light.

"I don't think Mabel will understand at all," she said as she examined the pieces in her hand. "I think she's going to hate me for a very long time."

## Chapter 12

Tim took the news in his typical fashion. He blew up. He was still ranting when Lois climbed the stairs to return to her room.

Mabel had disappeared earlier that morning with one of her friends. She wouldn't even speak to her sister. Lois related all of this to Seamus when he called her that afternoon.

"So, they all know," he said. "I suppose Dad blew a gasket."
"Yes, he did." She paused. "I think his attitude toward you might change though. I...I told Mom about what

happened when you were in Anaheim."

The silence was deafening. Her stomach twisted into a knot. "I'm sorry, Seamus, I know I shouldn't have said anything. But I couldn't let them think that way about you anymore. I didn't tell them anything else. I-"
"It's okay," he said. "Don't worry. I get it. I guess it had to come out sometime. How did your mom take it?"

"Mom was just mad because I didn't tell her right away," she said. "I think she'll be picking out the china pattern in the next few...Oh, God! You didn't hear that. Just disregard. Disregard!"

Seamus laughed. "Well, I have to go. My break is over and I don't think the boss will appreciate it if I start slacking on the first day. Especially with the mood he's in. The Billionaire may disown me after all this."
"He'll be sorry if he does. Call me later?"
"I will. I love you."

She smiled. "I love you too."
"Hey! Wait a minute!"
"Yes?"
"Is blue still your favorite color?"
"It is."

"Good." He ended the call.
A knock sounded on Lois's door. Thinking it might be Mabel, she rose and quickly opened it. Tim stood

outside.

"Can I come in?" he asked.
She nodded and stood aside so that he might enter.
He took a seat in the chair near her desk.
Tim looked as though he had lost his best friend. She
had never seen him look so defeated.

"Why didn't he tell me?" He wasn't looking at her
when he asked the question, so she wasn't sure
whether he was talking to her or to himself.

"He was only ten. He didn't know how."
"If I had known," he said, shaking his head. "I
would've killed that son of a—"
"Tim," she said gently. "I'm not the one you should be
saying this to."

He nodded. Then, for the first time, faced her.
"He just got off break," she said. "But, I think he'll talk
to the boss." She offered him the handset of her
telephone.
He took it and said, "You're sure?"
"Yes."

He accepted the handset.
Lois opened the door and stepped out into the hall.

**Chapter 13**

The next few months passed slowly, but they passed.

Lois kept busy at the antique store and talked to Seamus every day.  She saw nothing of Mabel.

As summer gave way to autumn, she became increasingly concerned about her sister. The tension between them had grown palpable, to the point that it seemed to be a separate entity in and of itself. The afternoon before Seamus's fight, a heavy fragrance of rain hung in the Autumn air.  Fat droplets streaked the windows by the time Cathy and Tim headed out for the evening, leaving the two girls alone in the house.

Lois was walking past Mabel in the second floor corridor when her sister veered into her, crashing her into the wall. Mabel had continued down the hall without another word.
Lois chased her down.

"What was that about?" She clamped a hand on her sister's shoulder and spun her around. They stood on the landing just above the stairs.
"I don't know what you're talking about," Mabel said icily.

"You damn well do! You just about threw me into the wall! Let's have it out now, Mabel. Stop avoiding and ignoring me."

Her sister's eyes turned to slits. "You knew how I felt about him!  How could you do what you did?  You said you didn't want him!"

"I didn't know this would happen, Mabel. I didn't expect it. I didn't mean it to hurt you, and I'm sorry. Can't we put it behind us? Why can't you understand? I want you and I to be friends again."

Mabel crossed her arms, resembling the child she had once been. She shook her head. "You are such a liar, Lois. All this time, you were scheming to get him. He was mine!"

"He isn't a toy." A slow rage began to fill her. She could feel it in the blood that thundered in her ears. "He wasn't interested in you anyway. He thought of you as a sister, nothing more."

Mabel suddenly attacked her. She grabbed hold of Lois's hair and tore at her clothes. Lois's foot connected with her shin and Mabel cried out in pain. She shoved Lois backward and she teetered on the edge of the stairs. She couldn't hold her balance. She fell.

Lois rolled, striking her head on the steps on the way down.
Mabel ran by her as she lay dazed near the bottom of the stairway. The door slammed and the girl was gone.

Lois shambled painfully to her feet. Nothing seemed

to be broken, but she was sure there would be bruises later. Her body wasn't what hurt most, though. Tears cascaded down her cheeks as she made her way back up the stairs.

Seamus answered on the first ring. He was in his car. Her voice dissolved into tears the minute he answered.
"Lois, I can't understand you. What happened?" he said.

"She hates me, Seamus!" The words came out in between sobs.
"Who?"
"Mabel. She pushed me —oh Seamus!"
"I'm on my way. Just stay put."

He arrived a few minutes later and called to her as he ascended the stairs. She waited in the bedroom.
His expression was grim when he looked at her. "My God...how did this happen?" he asked. He touched her arm where a large, purple contusion had blossomed.
"I must have gotten it when I fell down the stairs."
"You fell? Are you alright?"

"I think so. Just sore."
She was holding her head. He pulled her hand away and found a large bump.
 "Did Mabel do this?" he asked.

"We were fighting and I fell."

"You said she pushed you."

"I don't know. I...it's all my fault!" She broke down again.

"Get some things together," he said. "I'm taking you to my place."

"But—"

"I'll call Dad and Cathy. Just get ready to go."

"Don't tell them what happened," she pleaded.

He seemed not to hear her as he dialed.

Seamus held her hand as they drove to his apartment, squeezing it gently in time to the music on the radio. A weight seemed to lift from her the further they drove from the house.

"What did Mom say?" she asked.

"She said that Mabel called her a few minutes before I did, bawling her eyes out. She thought she killed you. Needless to say, she'll be glad you're alive."

"We should have stayed there then. She'll be alone in the house."

"She'll be fine. And she'll still be there tomorrow when I bring you home. Forget about her for now."

"But I'll distract you from the fight. Plus you need your sleep."

"I don't need sleep, I need you," he blurted out. "I should have had you there the whole time."

She lapsed into silence. He would get no more

argument from her.

When she arrived at his apartment, unfamiliar shadows greeted her. Seamus flipped a switch and her eyes took in the now furnished apartment.
"What do you think?" he asked.
The living room set was blue.

A lump formed in her throat. "I love it."
She threw her arms around him and kissed him.
He lifted her into his arms, cupping her bottom with both hands. The kiss deepened.

"We can't do anything," she warned. "I'll make your legs weak."
"You're right," he said as he carried her to the bedroom. He took her to the bed.

"Seamus, we can't! I'll make you weak!"
He didn't answer as he removed her blouse.
"Seamus, are you listening to me?"

He pulled her bra off, exposing her breasts. She leaned back so that he could remove her shoes, socks and jeans.
"Wait!" she said as he reached for the elastic of her panties. "Wait a minute!"

He paused. His eyes were feverish.
"I am more than happy to give you exactly what you want and more but, first, answer me one question. Is

this going to hurt your chances of winning the fight?"
"It could," he admitted.

"Then...maybe we should wait. I'll sleep with you tonight, but we won't do anything. Ok?"
He leaned back and let out a deep breath as he stared at the ceiling.

"I'll make it up to you tomorrow night. I promise."
"Ok," he grumbled.
"And maybe you had better stay dressed...just in case."

## Chapter 14

The rain pattered softly against the windows as Lois listened to the soft exhalation of Seamus's breath. He was fully dressed and facing away from her.
She had put her blouse back on, but that was all. When she was sure he was asleep, she scooted up against him and drifted off.

She awoke to a hand between her legs. Seamus had turned over. At first, she thought he was awake, but his soft snore in her ear convinced her otherwise. His hand was warm. She turned a little and realized that his lips were very close to her own. Her body began to tingle.

The hand began to move in lazy circles. Then it ceased. She glanced at him. He was still snoring.

The lazy circles started up again.
"Seamus?" she whispered.

His hand moved up to her stomach. It slid back down and caught the elastic of her panties, pulling them along with it.

Seamus's body began to shake a little. She leaned over to her bedside lamp and clicked the switch.
"You're awake!" she cried. "And you're laughing!"
He turned over and snickered

"That is not fair." she protested.
"What? I was sleeping..."
"You were not. You were turning me on!"
She climbed atop him, straddling him.
"Now, who's turning who on?" he said. He pulled her down and kissed her.

"I really don't want to ruin this for you," she moaned.
"Who says you will. Maybe you'll make me stronger."
She rose and pulled her shirt off. He cupped her breasts, twisting the nipples between his thumb and forefinger. She pulled away gasping.
"Where are they?"
"On the shelf. Above your head."

She pulled out a condom. Then moved to unbutton his jeans. She released and sheathed him, then she removed her panties.
When she gripped his member, it was like living stone

beneath her fingertips. She guided him in and sank down on the shaft. He was in deep and she gasped in delight.

Lois leaned forward as he bucked against her. Her nipples were near his lips and he caught them with his tongue as she rocked back and forth. The sensation awoke an unquenchable fire within her.

She cried out as the first of her orgasms peaked, then fell forward suddenly helpless. He did not allow her to recover.

Waves of pleasure exploded over her as the next ascent began. The friction they were producing seemed to be heating him within her. She whimpered. She rose up off of her knees and repositioned herself so that she was on her feet. Then, she dropped her hips so that she could take him even more deeply. He groaned.

"Are you ready?" she asked.
He never gave her an answer. She rose, turned to face his feet and began rocking again. He grasped hold of her hips.
"Oh...God!"

Her climax was growing as he spoke. Each word electrified her. She began to pant as a string of orgasms shook her body. Each sensation was like a bolt of electricity that left her trembling in anticipation of the next. She was dimly aware that he had joined her on that plateau.

She rolled off of him and he pulled her into his arms. They lay still for a bit, allowing the aftershocks of their passion to recede as their breathing returned to normal.
"I hope this won't hurt anything," she said.
"I told you, I think it'll make me stronger."
"Well, if it does work, we'll have to do it before every fight."

"Sounds good to me." he paused. "I forgot to tell you, I invited Dad and Cathy to the fight."
"That's wonderful! What did they say? Are they coming?"

"They are. My Dad actually sounded pretty pleased about it."
She touched the eye of the eagle. "Are you going to tell them everything?"

"One thing at a time," he said.
"Cora told me about it," she confessed. "Why did you cover the scars with tattoos?"
"Because I had to shoot back," he said. "And I don't miss."

## Chapter 15

Gulls danced in the sky as Seamus drove Lois back to

the house. They swept down in graceful arcs, bodies pale against the grey sky, harbingers of a coming storm.

"Don't worry now," Seamus said as they parted. "Everything will be fine."

He kissed her lips.

"I hope so," she said.

As she watched him go, someone stepped out of the front door and stood by her side.

"Lois?"

"Yes?"

Mabel's eyes were welling with tears. "I'm so sorry." Lois gathered her sister into her arms. She held her tightly. "It's ok, Sissy. I'm sorry too. I should have been honest with you but, at the time, I couldn't even be honest with myself."

"I feel so stupid," her sister said. "Mom and I talked. She made me see what I was doing."

"Mom is pretty good at that."

"And then Tim had a talk with me."

"Tim too, huh?"

"And one other person. I think he was the most convincing."

"He can be."

"He's a really great guy," she said. "But he really isn't really my type."

"Oh?"

"Well, he's not much of a bad boy, is he?"
Lois laughed as she put an arm around her. "I guess we'll see. Are you coming to his fight?"
"I sure am."

"Then we'd better get spruced up. And today, I won't even complain about what you have on."
"Good, because I have this really cute strapless dress I've been wanting to wear and I think you're going to love it!"

"I guess you'll have to show me."
"Come on and see."
Lois sighed.
***


They arrived shortly before fight time in Tim's Cadillac Escalade. The match was taking place at one of the better known casinos and parking was scarce. It took Tim a while to find a spot. When he finally did, Lois and Mabel hurried ahead.

The casino was buzzing with activity. They hurried through the gaming floor and up into the special area designated for large events. The place was packed. Lois spied Seamus through the red ropes surrounding the ring. When he saw her, he winked.

Seamus had already been introduced by the time they entered the room. The ring announcer was introducing the bald man she knew as Lead Head. Al beckoned them over to their seats.

"This is my sister, Mabel," Lois said by way of introduction.

"You're in for a real show," Al said with a grin. "Seamus is a bad ass in the ring." He gave Mabel an appreciative look. "Nice dress."

"Thanks!" she gushed.

Lead Head's name was actually Lloyd Hedstrom. He looked far more intimidating in the ring than he did in street clothes. The man was a mountain of muscle. Tim and Cathy joined them just as the bell rang.

A knot had been forming in Lois's stomach all day. The uncomfortable feeling had now wound its way into her throat. Nausea washed over her as a single question repeated itself like a mantra in her mind. What if I ruined him?

The two fighters approached one another and touched gloves. Lead Head, balanced on his toes threw a jab at Seamus's chin. He avoided it easily. The bald man's mouth seemed to be incessant. Lois wished she could read lips.

Seamus held his gloves up when another blow came toward his face. Lead Head forced him backward against the ropes. The crowd cheered.

Nick shouted to Seamus from his corner. "Fight back, Irish!"

Leah Head continued to pummel him.

"Oh, Seamus!" Lois breathed. She imagined his legs going out from under him. It would be her fault if he lost.

Lead Head's blows seemed to drop. They were so low, the referee had to step in and warn him. A chorus of "boos" filled the room.

They returned to the center of the ring.

While Seamus's hands were low, Lead Head stepped forward and cuffed his ear. Seamus stumbled.

Lois rose to her feet.

A dangerous darkness shone in Seamus's eyes. He planted his right foot and delivered a bone crushing blow to Lead Head's jaw with his right hand. His next blow came from the left as he drove his fist into Lead Head's mid-section. The boxer's eyes dilated as he fell to the mat. He lay there, stunned.

The referee counted, but Lead Head failed to stir. By the time he came to, the ref had reached ten. The official raised Seamus's hand above his head. The crowd cheered.

"Told you he was a bad ass," Al said.

Seamus came to the edge of the ring and stepped through the ropes. When he stepped down from the ring, she rushed to him.

"See?" he said. "It worked!"

"I guess we'll have to do that before every fight from now on."

"For the rest of my career at least. But how about the rest of our lives?"

"I am not going to assume on this one," she said. "I guess you'll have to spell it out for me."

"Marry me."

She threw her arms around him.

"I assume that's a yes."

"Assume away," she beamed, "assume away!"

## 8. The art of penetration.

Now, we are getting down to business. We already talked about oral sex. We already talked about setting the mood. We have even talked about the psychology of sex. Now, it is all about the in and outs, literally, of sex.

Most guys would really think about penetration simply as that: a quick in and out affair. You get in, take care of business, and get out. If you think this way, I don't blame you. That is how we are hardwired.

Well, you need to get that mindset out of your mind. If you want to be a good lover, you have to take care of your needs first. Penetration must serve both her and your interests. And, the interesting thing about effective and highly memorable sex is a lesson you need to learn in sales: the customer always comes first.

Your partner has to come first. I am not talking about just putting her needs first, but she has to physically climax first. Make her climax your top priority. You can come later. Otherwise, you are going to be a lousy lover, as far as she is concerned.

We all want to be invited back to the party.

<u>Penetration techniques.</u>

There are many ways to penetrate a woman.

It may seem like there is only one way, which is to put your dick in there, thrust forward, and keep repeating it until you come. Well, that is true. But there are many different ways to do it.

<u>Speed.</u>

Ideally, you should have 3 modes: orgasm mode, slow and steady, and intermediate rhythm. A great technique is to mix these 3 modes up continually, so she is always getting something new and the penetration doesn't get stale and boring.

I am sorry to break it to you, but a jackhammer style of fucking is not necessarily welcome all the time. It all depends on context. If you are leading up with your honey, for a quick 15 minute bang during her lunch break, banging her like a jackhammer makes all the sense in the world.

However, if you just watched a movie or a play together, or had a nice romantic dinner at a five star restaurant, a jackhammer approach probably doesn't fit the whole motif and theme of the evening. You might want to match your penetration speed with the mood.

Now, what is important here is that you need to mix up your speed. You have to pay attention to where she is, in terms of climaxing, and match her speed. The secret to women is that they start out slow. It really takes a long time to warm the oven, as far as women are concerned.

Ramp it up, and once you notice that she is getting heated, then you turn up the speed and give it to her.

Angles.

There are different angles that you can take. You can lean to the right or left to hit the sides of her vaginal wall, or you can position yourself so that you are rubbing against her clitoris whenever you thrust. You can also penetrate her in a downward motion (in missionary), so her vaginal wall (the one she shares with her anus) is getting a lot of stimulation.

One of the best ways to do this is, of course, to change the angle of your penis. When you are in there, you need to move around. Move your butt around. Try to form the letters of the alphabet when you are thrusting in and out. You would be surprised as to the kind of feedback you would get.

Pay attention to how she is moaning. If you notice a certain changes in how she is moaning, you would realize that you are hitting a very sensitive spot. Repeat that. You might want to do some more teasing, or change the speed. But you need to repeat that, because you might be on to something.

The secret to effective and highly enjoyable sex positions, of course, is the angle of your penis. That is the whole point behind sex positions, in the first place. Different positions involve different angles of thrusting and penetration. Play around with the angles, to find her G-spot and to fully engage her

Your hands.

Don't just leave them on her legs, holding them apart. Put her legs on your shoulders, spread them way apart, or put her feet on your chest. Grab her breasts while you are penetrating her. Grab her hips pull her towards you. Put your finger inside her mouth and tell her to suck it like a cock. There are endless possibilities, but just remember to use your hands to your benefit in extra stimulation for her.

Teasing.

You can tease a woman with your dick.

Many guys forget about this. They just thrust it in, and leave it in. No. You can tease her, really. You can rub against her clit, which most women dig. You can wiggle around her vaginal cavity. You can slide your penis to the sides of her pussy. Thrust in halfway for a minute, then slam your whole cock inside her, which will surprise and excite her.

The key here is to get her excited. The key here is to tease her and not just jam it in. You know you are doing a good job when she begs you to stick it in. Make it a point to tease her until she begs you to stick it in.

## 9. Seven positions for her maximum pleasure.

It is very easy for guys to think that all sexual positions are intended and designed primarily for men. live in a male-centered world. As much progress as we have made in terms of gender equality, old mental habits die hard. This is especially true when it comes to sex.

It is easy for guys to pick and choose sexual positions primarily based on how easy it would be for them to get off. This is a bad move if you are trying to impress a woman sexually. Remember, if you want to be a better lover, she has to come first.

You need to make her pleasure a priority if you want to get invited back to the party. If you want her to have a very favorable impression of you, both as a romantic and a sexual partner, you have to make her needs top priority. Instead of automatically picking sexual positions that favor you, focus on what is pleasurable for her.

Here are nine positions that maximize pleasure for her. The good news is that, the internet being the internet, there are tons of research materials you can check out, when looking into these positions. Many of these research resources have photos, so you don't have to scratch your head as to what these positions look like. There are more than enough resources out there to help you pull off these sexual positions like a pro.

Standing.

It is all about positioning. The great thing about sex while standing is that there is a lot of emotional urgency to it.

Usually, people who have sex standing are those people who don't have much time to get off. There is this sense of danger. There is this sense of surprise. There is that improvised atmosphere to the air when you are doing it while standing up.

While, physically speaking, this does not necessarily get her off, it does, psychologically, get her excited. Since sex is 90% psychological and 10% physical, this position definitely deserves to be at the top of the list.

Doggie style.

Doggie style is pretty straightforward. It is one of the most basic sexual positions. It is also one of the most effective and popular. The reason why it is very popular is because it pleasures both men and women.

It allows for maximum clitoral stimulation, especially if you reach over her hips and rub her clit from behind. It also maximizes vaginal penetration. Whether you are trying to get your partner to orgasm through stimulating her clitoris, or you want to get her off by exciting her G-spot, doggie style is it. Also, doggie style isn't very complicated. You don't have to be a rocket scientist to pull this off.

Cowgirl.

Cowgirl position is pretty straightforward. The woman straddles the man while he is flat on his back. The great thing about the cowgirl position is that it maximizes control for the woman.

To orgasm, women have a certain pattern and rhythm. They need to build up slowly, and then pick up pace and scale. Guys sometimes completely lose sight of this fact and, eventually either pump too hard, pump too slow, or do something that prevents the woman from climaxing. You can get her close to it, but it only takes a few missteps and the opportunity closes.

When you allow a woman to straddle you cowgirl style, she can control her orgasm. It would be a very pleasurable experience for both of you. The cowgirl position involves her facing you so there is that added element of intimacy.

Spooning.

If you think that it is romantic to lie down at the back of

your partner and cuddle, you will find spooning sex very sexy. This is because it has the emotional intimacy of spooning while you are penetrating her.

The same applies to your partner. Your partner feels appreciated, loved, caressed, and sexually gratified. Again, this is primarily psychological because, in terms of clitoral contact, spooning is kind of a difficult position, to maximize clitoral or G-spot contact. It does happen, though.

Sideways cowgirl.

This is for the more athletic women out there. Cowgirl and reverse cowgirl positions are pretty straightforward because you are basically just sitting on your partner's penis. However, sideways cowgirl involves the woman sitting at a 90 degree angle to her partner. Instead of straddling him straight on, she sits to the side.

The great about the sideways cowgirl is that it increases clitoral stimulation and maximizes control, because the woman is still on top. It does take a lot more effort to perfect. But, if you are looking for your female partner to come regularly and predictably, this is the position you should encourage her to take. It takes an adventurous woman to try this because it does take quite a bit of effort.

Sitting face to face.

If you are looking for a lot of intimacy, if you are sexually adventurous and you want to create a really sexy environment, you may want to try sitting face to face while having sex. This position is between cowgirl and mission.

What happens is you start in cowgirl and have the girl riding you. Then you sit up and hold her close with your arms. There may not be much motion or thrusting, but it is more of a position to make sex highly romantic, highly personal, and very very emotionally intimate.

It takes a while to come in this position, for both men and women.

Missionary.

This is like the plain vanilla sexual position. It seems like almost anybody knows how to do this. You will be just completely clueless about your body if you don't even know how missionary position looks like. Interestingly enough, missionary position actually maximizes pleasure for the woman on both the psychological and physical level.

Physically, it is fairly easy to see why this stimulates women, because you are essentially just lying right on top of her clitoris. You only need to thrust in the right angle to get her excited. You only need to adopt the right speed and rhythm to match her normal cycle for orgasms.

Missionary enables women to orgasm multiple times because it delivers on two levels. First, it maximizes clitoral stimulation and paves the way for G-spots stimulation. Also, since you are looking at each other face to face, you can kiss each other, caress each other, and really be in each other's intimate space, psychological intimacy is also present.

This is also the best position to whisper naughty nothings to each other in, and if you combine all of the following with strong eye contact, then she will never be wetter.

As I keep saying, sex is 90% psychological and emotional, and 10% physical. Missionary position delivers on both.

## 10. Orgasms 101.

Now, we are getting to the good stuff. We are talking about the ultimate destination: the promised land of sex in the eyes of many men.

Most men would look at sex as primarily a physical, or even mechanical, series of actions leading to the promised land, or promised outcome of orgasm. Never ever overlook the fact that if you want your partner to orgasm, you cannot neglect the emotional and psychological factor involved in orgasm.

Sex is a holistic experience. It is not just a physical reaction of your lower central nervous system.

It is not just your body doing something because your nerves were stimulated enough. A key component of that overall stimulation is how you feel, how comfortable you are, how adventurous you are, your emotional intensity, and other factors that involve your emotions and mind.

As I keep mentioning in this book, sex is 90%

psychological and emotional, and 10% physical.

We tend to look at sex as primarily a physical phenomenon. But, make no mistake about it. Sex involves all of you. It is no surprise that many traditions, both philosophical and spiritual, tie sex in with a higher state of being. You only need to look at Hinduism and Tantra to see how sex, as an act, is linked to higher states of consciousness and spiritual awakening.

With this frame of mind, orgasms should not just be looked at as a base physical reaction. If you want a truly meaningful orgasm for both you and your partner, you have to look at it as a way to express not just your physical attraction, but also the depth of your love and your emotional intensity.

Clitoral or vaginal orgasm?

There are more ways to make a woman come than just rubbing her magic button. Clitoral stimulation is not the only game in town, as far as orgasms are concerned.

Unfortunately, popular media and popular culture has made many guys think that the only way women really come is through clitoral stimulation. While this is true for the vast majority of women, the fact is, relatively few women experience vaginal orgasms. And that's okay. Not everyone can do it, and you shouldn't feel disappointed or make them feel judged if they don't.

Make her squirt.

Did you know that women ejaculate just like guys? I am not talking about urine here. I am talking about a clear odorless liquid that women are capable of expelling. Just as men ejaculate semen when they orgasm, women can squirt as well.

I know you are probably rolling your eyes or scratching your head. You might even think that this is just an urban legend that has been perpetrated and popularized by pornography. The reality is that it is true. This is a scientifically documented fact. Women can be made to squirt. This is the highest form of orgasm for women.

Usually, when women come, they just make a lot of noise. Sometimes, their eyes go back to the back of their heads, their toes curl, and they exhibit lots of physical signals. But that is circumstantial evidence that they came. A lot of those signals can be faked.

If you really want to know whether you hit a home run or not, try to make her squirt. Squirting orgasms are normally achieved through a combination of clitoral and vaginal, or G-spot stimulation. It will take quite a bit of time.

One of the best ways to do it is to go down on her for quite some time, to really heat her up to a high enough level. Know what kind of sexual positions she prefers the most. Then you need to stimulate her G-spot a lot, intensely, and much harder than you think you would with two fingers.

You will insert your fingers and curl them towards you in a "come here" sign, which rubs them against her G-spot. You'll know you're doing it right if you hear what sounds like liquid splashing around inside of her.

Making your woman squirt is a great goal to have, because the focus is on her. It is not on you ejaculating. It is on her; you're not even being touched. The more you please her, the more she will please you.

Make her speechless.

Orgasm is an aural experience. If it is done right and achieved properly, there is no need for words. It becomes an almost mystical experience that leaves your woman speechless. Aim for that.

Multiple orgasms.

Multiple orgasms are a distinct gift given by nature to women. I am sorry, guys, but we are just not typically capable of multiple orgasms. The great thing about multiple orgasms is that, if you are able to stimulate your woman to an intense first orgasm, you can switch things up to make her come again.

For example, if you have made your woman come through clitoral stimulation, you can switch to vaginal stimulation or G-spot stimulation, to make her come again. Once she comes that way, you can then switch back to clitoral stimulation. You can keep playing this game again and again, and see how many times you can make her orgasm. This is just a distinct gift women have, that guys don't.

## 11. Anal sex.

Now, we are getting a little bit down and dirty.

Anal sex is not welcomed by all women.

There is a difference between your woman sitting down with you watching a few porn movies off the internet involving anal sex, and you packing her fudge. There oftentimes a clear divide between fantasy and reality.

If you want to try anal sex with your woman, you have approach it in a very careful way. You have to, obviously, get her consent.

The secret to pulling this off is to cater to her curiosity.

The interesting thing about anal sex is that it is very different from male anal sex. It is very easy to understand why anal sex is very popular with guys who are receiving it, because the male prostate is loaded with nerves.

When a man comes by penetrating somebody, only part

of those nerves are engaged. When the backside of the prostate is engaged, coupled with the man stimulating his penis, male orgasm is complete. This is why many men who receive anal sex are addicted to that form of sex because, according to research studies, it gives them a "fuller" form of male orgasm.

Obviously, women don't have prostates, so full orgasms from anal sex is not possible with them. So, what can they possibly get from it since they don't have the equipment to come from anal sex? As I keep mentioning in this book, sex is 90% psychological and emotional, 10% physical.

This is definitely at play when it comes to anal sex. Even though the woman isn't physically equipped to come from anal sex, there is still enough nerve stimulation that can feed into the emotional and psychological urgency of doing something nasty and forbidden and taboo.

Anal sex has been forbidden in many spiritual, philosophical and cultural traditions throughout history. In fact, it is banned by many cultures. There is something inherently adventurous about it, because it is forbidden.

This is just the same way people seek out drugs. If you forbid something, people will find it adventurous, and would do it. Anal sex is one of those sexual practices.

That is its appeal to women. That sense of danger, mystery, rebelliousness, and the thrill of doing something you aren't supposed to do, impacts female psychology.

When paired with the nerve stimulation, as well as your overall stimulation of her body or breasts, her face or hair, it can lead to an emotional rush.

This is not a physical orgasm. As I have mentioned, there such a thing as a mental and emotional stimulation. It get definitely get her off, at least, on an emotional level. So, how do you get your woman to do this? How do you prepare your woman for this?

Mental preparation.

Proper preparation must first start with getting your woman comfortable. You have to appeal to her sense of curiosity. You have to appeal to her sense of mystery.

Raise it as a joke, from time to time. At first, she may respond negatively. She might even be offended. But, if you raise it in enough number of times, you might break her down a bit and appeal to her sense of curiosity. All you are doing is planting the seed in her mind with this.

You will be able to gauge her reaction to your joke to see how open she is to it. You will sometimes need to be patient, and it might not even be in the cards for you ever. This is okay.

Now, if you are able to get her to give you permission to do this, make sure it is extremely pleasurable to her. Otherwise, it is going to be a one-time event for you.

Make sure she knows the pleasure she will be getting from it, and make it about pleasing her and exploring something together, as opposed to focusing on your own desires.

If she has any interest in it, she will make it known once you bring it up and let her know that you won't be judging her for it!

Physical preparation.

Physical preparation is pretty straightforward.

Get her in the mood. Get her excited. Get her psychologically and emotionally in the same place you are in.

You should also look into a small buttplug for her. This is for her to wear for a series of hours – anywhere from 1-4 hours before the deed – to make sure that she is stretched adequately, and that your cock will not prove too sudden of a painful penetration. This part is key to making sure that she doesn't experience much pain, and that it is mutually pleasurable.

By using a buttplug she can also envision your cock inside her asshole for hours, which will turn her on to no end.

Hygiene.

Hygiene is obviously a large concern when it comes to

anal sex.

If all you see is the final product, and you are led to believe that anal sex is nice and clean. It is anything but. So if you want to prepare your partner properly for anal sex, you need to go the whole nine yards. You need to talk to her about what you both need to do, so she is ready for it.

This is very important because it impacts smell and it impacts what you see. It also impacts the cleanliness of the sheets and the place you are going to have anal sex in. So, hygiene is extremely important.

Luckily, it's far easier than you think it would be. There are just three steps you need to take for flawlessly clean anal sex.

First, make sure that your woman has a bowel movement within a few hours before you plan to have anal sex. This will make sure that you don't get any surprises, and that her anus is empty of fecal matter for the most part. This gets rid of 90% of the worry with anal sex. Also related to this point is to make sure that she doesn't eat spicy or volatile food that might cause her to have diarrhea within 1-2 days before you plan the act. This is a good idea for obvious reasons.

Second, have her do an enema a couple of hours before you plan to have anal sex. For those that don't know, an enema is a sort of spout that you pour into your anus that irrigates and cleans it. The main use is to clean the anus for colonoscopies, but this is obviously a very valid use as well. This will eliminate the last 10% of fecal matter from the anus, making your gal sparkling clean.

Finally, baby wipe her bum. Use a scented baby wipe to wipe around any excess liquid or matter that might be around her anus. This will make her asshole smell nice and fresh, and maybe even inviting to you.

Technique.

You have to be very gentle, especially if your partner is an anal sex virgin. You need to make sure that you are properly lubricated not just on your penis, but you also have to lubricate her anus – it does not self-lubricate like her pussy. Too many guys make the rookie mistake that, as long as they put enough lube on their junk, they are good to go.

This is absolutely wrong. The lube moves backwards, and it might still be a rough experience for your partner. So, make sure that she is lubed up as well.

You need to start slow. Pay attention to how she is moving. If you notice that she is supporting her open palms against your legs, that is a sign. It means that you are going too fast too hard. Try to read her body language, to basically have her guide you into it.

You have to remember, when you are doing anal sex with

a woman, you are trying to please her because you want her to do this again. If you are doing anal sex just to please yourself, you are doing it wrong. This is going to be a one-time event. So, pay careful attention to your technique. Don't hit her hard from the back like a jackhammer. That is not going to work.

Build it up slowly. Make sure that she is emotionally engaged. Kiss her from the back. Kiss the back of her neck. Be gentle with her, and really create a deeply emotionally intimate moment. This way, she feels that she is doing something risky, but at the same time she feels reassured, confident, and loved.

That is the key. Make her feel appreciated. Make her feel special in your space together. It is not about you and your pleasure. It is about you together, exploring a new sexual horizon.

And in that vein, make sure to mention that it's dirty, hot, and arousing. This will encourage her to keep going, turn her on, and remind her of the sexy reasons she is engaging in it.

Finally, condoms. Since the anus does not self-lubricate, it is prone to microtears in the skin – of course, this is essentially whats leads the the transmission of STDs. So sticking with condoms is the wise move, as well as not ejaculating into the anus for similar reasons.

## 12. Getting kinky.

We have already covered the ins and outs of mostly normal sex. Now, we are going to dial it up a notch. I am going to talk about kinky sex.

Why do people put on vinyl or leather, and allow their partner to tie them up, slap them around and whip them? Why do people like to be dominated sexually? Why do couples engage in swapping partners? The answer is simple. In fact, the answer in this book keeps coming up again and again.

Sex is 90% psychological and emotional, 10% physical.

Kinky sex is really all about the psychological and emotional components of sex. Kinky sex is all about the environment, the atmosphere, the ambiance and the emotional intensity of the moment.

Don't get me wrong. There are certain people with psychological conditions, namely masochism, who get off on pain. But aside from that, there is a distinct psychological thrill that many otherwise normal people get from doing something they feel they shouldn't be doing. Novelty and naughtiness rule the day.

Society has many conventions and norms. Many people get off sexually when violating these norms. The psychological and emotional component is very high, while the physical component is pretty straightforward. The sex involved in BDSM, domination, and swinging are quite conventional. It is the atmosphere that people are looking for. It is that mental rush that they are after.

Here is just an overview of the many kinky practices you might want to consider, depending on what you are into.

Blindfold, tying up and BDSM.

Blindfolding your partner and trying her up, or being blindfolded, tied up and dominated by your partner, all flow from the same place. They all flow from the thrill of doing something dangerous, risky and mysterious – all while handing control over to someone else.

People who are into BDSM don't make a big deal out of what they are doing. They don't publicly go out there and say, "Yes, I dress up in all leather and vinyl. Let myself be tied down and have a woman in stockings and garters, with her tits hanging out, beat the heck out of me." People aren't normally that open about that aspect of their lives.

This is precisely why BDSM, blindfolding, or tying up is so kinky to many people. It is because there is that secret life dynamic going on. They feel this spices up their sex life.

The aspect of control is also underrated. It's a feeling that your life and pleasure is completely in someone else's hands, and they must trust you. This is the arousing part of blindfold, tying up, and BDSM for most. This goes for both the controller, AND the controlled party.

The controller likes to be in charge and dictate exactly what happens in their sexual encounters, while the controlled likes to be told what to do and exactly how to do it. Some just like to be in charge, while some like to be led and not think about it.

If you blindfold or tie up your partner, make sure that the binds aren't too tight, and they can actually escape at any moment if they choose to. The blindfolds and ties are actually symbolic, and shouldn't serve to actually restraint them against their wills.

If you are tying your girl up, I would suggest tying their hands in front of their body as opposed to behind, because that way she can still touch you somewhat. Also, it's very easy for hands tied behind the body to become uncomfortable and cramp, and she will also have difficulty switching positions and such.

Choking, slapping and domination.

The interesting thing about the domination sexual subculture is that a high proportion of otherwise powerful men are into it. These are bankers, lawyers, or captains of industry - you know, pillars of society.

They then allow themselves to be submissive, often cold, naked on the floor, and bound up with a ball gagging their mouth. Then, a woman in vinyl, partly nude or fully clothed, whipping them.

What gives?

Guys who are into this sexualize the reversal of power roles. In the normal world, they are on top of the world. They call the shots. These guys are the ones who make things happen. They have the money and the power to make things happen.

But, deep down, they find it attractive to reverse that role, to turn that world upside down and put a sexual spin to it. This is why there are many women who make a healthy living becoming dominatrix.

A large number of dominatrix, maybe even over 50%, don't even have sexual contact with their clients. They are just cracking the whip and, in many cases, beating their clients: stepping all over them and physically dominating them. The physical domination is what gets the man off. This is kinky. It is definitely unconventional. And, that is exactly why popular within a certain subculture of people.

When I say slapping by the way, I mean slapping in the face. Obviously, this is something you should make 100% sure that she wants, and then ask for feedback continually as to how hard you can do it.

This is doubly true for choking, as choking can actually render someone unconscious and is inherently dangerous. Put your hand at the base of her neck and try to spread out the pressure of your hand evenly on her neck. Then squeeze the neck a little bit, and apply pressure onto her neck. Go slowly so that you can both realize what her limits are, and the difference between turning her on and knocking her out.

When you get to be a pro at slapping and choking, you can combine them with fucking for extra, added effect.

Mutual masturbation.

There are people who get off on mutual masturbation. They don't want to have sex with each other. They just want to masturbate in front of another person who is also masturbating.

You are getting off in front of a woman who is getting herself off. And, this whole experience gets both of you off. The whole point here is psychological in nature.

You engage in mutual masturbation because the appeal is in "you can look, but don't touch". There is this psychological cat-and-mouse game. There is also this forbidden fruit theme to this.

It is really almost all psychological, because the physical component is you jerking yourself off. It is very straightforward, as far as the physical payoff for you is concerned. The big payoff for guys who are looking for this is primarily psychological and emotional. There is that thrill of the lack of sexual attainment that really gets people off.

The same applies to your partner. Your female partner must also get off on the whole mystique of being sexually stimulated without having direct physical contact. This is one of the highest levels of psychological sex games - mutual masturbation.

Swinging.

I have saved the most interesting for last. The most interesting kink, of course, is when you agree with your partner to have sex with another couple. And, that other couple agrees to swap partners with you. You would be surprised as to how popular swinging is.

Isn't the whole point of getting married becoming sexually exclusive to each other? Isn't that how loyalty and faithfulness are defined? Actually, these questions are the answers. People who are into swinging get turned on by the fact that they are redefining or violating traditional definitions of faithfulness and loyalty.

The key to successful swinging, of course, is to divorce the emotional component of your sexual relationship from the physical component. When you ask couples who have been married for a long time, and who are into swinging, one conclusion appears again and again.

They consider themselves 100% faithful to their partners even though they are swinging. They can effectively separate physical sensations from their love for their partner.

This can only happen when you successfully separate sexual exclusivity from emotional exclusivity.

Swinging has been around forever. What is new is that scientific studies of these sexual behaviors that started in the 1940s. But, if you were to look at ancient Greek pottery or Babylonian sculptures, this has been around forever.

Of course, different cultures have different attitudes regarding swinging. But, it is not going away anytime soon because of the psychological payoffs it has for the people who are into it.

A couple types of swinging are a mutual swap of both partners, and a swap of one partner while the other watches.

This is not dissimilar to an open relationship in many

ways, except open relationships can often lead to actual love interests.

## 13. Indulge some fantasies.

Sex can easily become mechanical and routine.

Sex can easily become an automatic physical series of actions.

The danger with looking at sex this way is that it becomes harder and harder to great sex. Can you come? Absolutely, especially if you are a man. You could do it automatically, each and every time. That is not the problem.

The problem is the quality of the experience - the depth of the intimacy that you are sharing with your partner. If you want sex to be something special instead of just something you do to pass the time or something you feel obligated doing so you can get off, you need to highlight the mental and emotional components of sex.

This is where fantasies come in.

If you are not into kinky sex, and many people aren't,

delivering on a fantasy can give them the missing elements that kinky sex often delivers. Whether you are looking for a sense of danger, a sense of mystery, emotional urgency, or a downright nasty element of spice in your lovemaking, fantasies can bring all that, and more, to the table.

Here are just some ways to engage the fantasy element of your sex life.

Dress up.

You would be surprised as to how much more pleasurable and exciting your partner would find sex if you dress up like a sailor, a soldier, or a cop. It is amazing. The same way, you would get more turned on or excited if your woman dressed up like a nurse or even just in sexy lingerie and a corset.

I am not talking about modern nurses with their ugly looking scrubs. I am talking about classic nurses, you know, with the white hat, with the red cross on top. Then, pair that up with garters, stockings and crotchless panties, and you got yourself a hot nurse fantasy. There is also the schoolteacher fantasy, and so on and so forth.

Never underestimate the power of uniforms. Uniforms bring up all sorts of emotional triggers that can really spice up your sex life. Dressing up doesn't just involve uniforms. There are many other ways you can dress up. You can dress up like a gorilla, or a teddy bear. Anything that is designed to get your partner excited is fair game, as far as costumes are concerned.

The idea is just to indulge your partner in something that they have always liked or wanted.

Role-play.

Role play is closely tied to dressing up in costumes.

Role-playing is all about capturing a certain ambience when you are having sex. Are you looking for a little bit of danger? Are you looking for a little bit of excitement due to something going wrong? Are you looking for some sort of imminent threat that can lead to a high level of emotional urgency?

That is what role-playing is all about. It is all about stepping into a role and soaking up the emotional atmosphere that role brings to the table. Also, there is a slight sense that you are doing something wrong, if you role-play, that would otherwise involve the law.

For example, you would be going to jail if you are a teacher and you have sex with your underage students. That is a no-brainer, right? Now, if you are with your partner who is 18 or above, you can role-play that you are a high school teacher and she is your student. The same sense of danger is still there, but nobody is going to get hauled off to jail.

That is the whole point of role-playing. It is trying to capture that sense of danger, the sense that you are doing something forbidden, but doing it within the safe legal confines of sex with somebody who can legally consent... but also something that you have always just fantasized about.

If you had a sexy teacher, the above might work. But the same applies if you have a sexy barista you see constantly, or have always loved men in police uniforms.

Also, role-play can involve playing roles of people you can't normally have sex with. You can pretend to be Bill Clinton and your partner could be Monica Lewinsky. That is what role-playing is. It is all about mentally transporting and transforming yourself to a place or to a role that you normally don't have.

Exhibitionism.

Some people get off on danger. There is something inherently exciting, to some people, about being found having sex in public. They get off on the thrill of being found out, or the risk of being found out. This makes sex more exciting. This makes sex more emotionally urgent.

You have to remember, the people who are exhibitionists or the people who have sex in public aren't doing it for their health. They are doing it to capture some sort of psychological and emotional payoff. They are not doing it primarily just to have sex. If they are looking just to physically get off and ejaculate or orgasm, they can do that indoors.

What they are looking for is a psychological or emotional orgasm that they can only get if they feel that there is a danger that they can go to jail, or people will ridicule them, or people would stop and look at point. That possibility is what gets them off. It's an incredibly thrill, and gets your adrenaline pumping like nothing else.

Threesomes.

Be honest, now. If you are a guy and you are reading this book, I am sure at least one time in your life, the thought has crossed your mind: of you having sex with your female partner and then her female friend, or maybe even her sister, joins in on the fun. It is OK to come clean, guys. This is a healthy male fantasy.

You are not a typical red blooded hetero-male if you haven't had at least a fantasy of having sex with more than one female at the same time. Threesomes are a very common fantasy, and some guys are able to successfully talk their female partner into allowing another female partner to join in on the fun.

The whole point into engaging in threesomes is, once again, not primarily physical, but psychological. It is not normal to have sex with more than one partner at the same time. Either a woman with two men, or a guy with two women, is just not conventional. So, that sense of violating conventionality or doing something you are not supposed to be doing is what adds spice to sex.

For the women, on the other hand, what they get out of it a sense of curiosity and a sense of danger, that they are doing something they shouldn't be doing. It is definitely an interesting fantasy, and a very common one at that. The hard reality is that most guys don't get to entertain that fantasy, unless of course they are having sex with two sex workers.

Force or rape fantasies.

We are getting a little bit serious here.

As I have mentioned earlier, role-playing allows you to engage in sexual behaviors that you might normally be able to engage in legally otherwise. The example that I gave was of a schoolteacher having sex with an underage student.

The same logic applies to force or rape fantasies. However, this is very different because you have to make sure that you and your partner are on the same page. You can't have a rape fantasy if your partner isn't into it. This can lead to real legal consequences for you.

Sex must always be about consent. It doesn't matter whether you are married to a person or not, or whether that person is a sex worker or not, that person must always consent. That is why it is really important, if you have a forced sex or rape fantasy, that your partner goes along.

There are some men who have this fantasy, but usually it is women who have this. So, make sure both of you are on the same page before you do this. Usually, force or rape fantasies all involve role-playing: she would be in the house, all alone; there would be a sense of danger because you would have to break in; and catch her by surprise. That kind of thing.

The whole appeal of it for a woman is to be dominated and lose control of herself to someone else. Obviously, this can't happen with you because you would never do such a thing – so how do you actually play out a rape fantasy? It's actually very simple.

You just act like you don't know her, tell her exactly what to do, and be a bit more forceful than you would otherwise. Just HOW forceful depends entirely on how much she goes along with the fantasy – if she seems like she is hesitant, then you probably have the green light to be more forceful and dominate her more.

Come in her mouth or on her face.

It seems obligatory in fuck films for the guy to pull out and ejaculate on the woman's face, or come in her mouth. It seems that it is not enough for a guy to pull out and come all over her stomach. He has to get up close and personal and just come on her face.

From a sociological, anthropological and psychological level, this puts a personal stamp on the orgasm. It is kind of a form of branding, if you are a cowboy. You have put your mark on her, and marked her as your territory. It's fairly personal, and not all women will enjoy it. Thus, this is something that you must make sure to ask for before sex, or during sex before your orgasm.

You may get a better reception if you ask during sex when she is in the mood to please you.

Then, all you have to do is remember to tell her right before you orgasm so she can prepare herself for you – mouth or face.

This also has elements of domination, which is the same reason that some women will refuse it. They think that coming on someone's face can be demeaning and embarrassing for women. Which, if you think about it, makes complete sense. So don't be upset if she refuses it, or refuses to swallow your come, which has the same elements of domination and degradation.

## 14. How to last longer and stay harder.

No one can be rock hard 100% of every sexual encounter. It doesn't matter how much of a sexual superstar you are. Sometimes we all go limp, prematurely ejaculate, or just malfunction. It happens to the best of us.

If you want to be the best lover you could be, sex has to be about both of you. You have to take care of her needs, and going limp certainly doesn't do that.

Here are some ways you can, not only last longer in the sack, but also stay harder and come right after she cums.

Do Kegel exercises daily.

Do you remember the time when you had to pee like a racehorse, but you had to hold it in? Do you remember the time when you were driving and you felt the need to urinate, but you can't find a gas station with a bathroom so you had to hold it in? Well, the skills you learned holding it in can really pay off.

When you are preventing yourself from peeing, you are exercising muscles in your groin area, that can come in handy when it comes to sex. Just as you can hold in urine with these exercises, you can prevent premature ejaculation. That is right. You can hold in your orgasm long enough for your partner to come.

When you flex that muscle for a few sets of 20 a day, you will be able to control your orgasm essentially. When you feel the orgasm bubbling up, you will simply be able to flex your kegels, and keep it at bay.

This is why male porn stars hang on to their job for such a long time. They can manage their ejaculation. Men have a better ability of doing this than women.

When you have such strong kegels, it also gives you harder, and higher quality erections because you literally have the ability to pump blood into your penis at will.

Avoid porn.

If you want to last longer in bed, if you want to stay harder and come much later, you only need to do one thing. I am sorry to break this to you, but porn has really ruined sex for many guys.

You might think that porn is a great quick and cheap way to get off. The internet, after all, is flooded with full length porn videos. The problem is, once you have a live female in front of you and you are doing it, all that porn can really get to your head.

Porn screws up your expectations. When you watch porn and you get off on porn, you are training yourself to get off based on your schedule. The problem is, when you have a real live female in front of you and you are having sex with her, you have to get off based on each other's schedule.

Sex is no longer about you. Porn is all about you. Porn is sex on demand, because you are having sex with yourself. To last longer in bed, and become a better lover, you need to get off porn totally. Maybe, put yourself on a porn diet for several weeks, if not months. You would be surprised as to how well your sex life improves.

Besides the psychological ghost of porn hanging over your real life sexual encounters, there is a very real physical difference between masturbating and real sex. Most of the time when men masturbate to porn, they are gripping their penis quite hard and tightly with their hand.

Obviously, a real vagina does not come close to the intensity of a death grip with your hand, so your penis may be desensitized and you may find it difficult to orgasm from a vagina alone.

Getting off porn and subsequently frequent masturbation will solve this, and make your penis more sensitive again.

Masturbate once a week.

I know this might sound like a contradiction to the advice I just gave without porn, but it makes sense. When you masturbate once a week **without** the aid of porn, you can feel more in control of your body. At the very least, you feel more aware of the patterns and signals your body sends out.

By being aware of the signals your body sends out, you can then mentally override them. You can stimulate yourself in such a way that you can come longer. Also, you can stimulate yourself in such a way that you can stay harder longer.

Masturbating once a week without the aid of porn is all about achieving a higher level of sexual self-awareness. Be in touch with what truly excites you, and form the right mental images so you can drag out ejaculation longer. The big payoff here is that the better you are at this, the more intense your climaxes are.

If you are like the typical guy, you would think that the sooner you come, the better. You are basically just settling for crumbs. Why settle for crumbs when you can have a nice cake?

The best way to do that is to pay more attention to yourself when you are masturbating, so you can psychologically condition yourself for a very very intense and full orgasm.

Take performance enhancers.

Performance enhancers are chemical aids that can help you last longer and prevent premature ejaculation. Most people would think that this involves viagra. But, I am talking about more than Viagra here.

There are herbal supplements you can take such as yohimbe and horny goat weed. Regardless, they all work the same way. They help dilate your blood vessels so enough blood gets into your equipment, so you stay harder for a longer period of time.

There are also performance enhancers you can take, that increase nerve stimulation of your orgasm so that, when you come, it is like having your mind blown open and seeing and experiencing the world with a brand new pair of eyes. You know that you have reached a high level of orgasm when the hairs all over your body rise up.

## 15. Sex toys 101.

You have to remember that if you want sex to be a truly meaningful experience for both you and your partner, you have to do whatever it takes.

You shouldn't say to your partner that if she wants to get off, she must only get off with the aid of your dick. If you want to restrict yourself to that situation, your sex life will suffer.

A lot of people talk about sex in glowing and reverent terms. But sometimes it is not this earth-shattering and ground-moving experience that many people paint it out to be. What is going on?

You might not be creating a full sexual experience.

You might want to look at sex the way you would when putting on a play or a production. All the elements have to be properly controlled and choreographed. Only when everything is in play and in place can you achieve the fullest effect. One way to do this is through the use of sex toys.

For her: vibrators, dildos, beads, clamps, whips, blindfolds, ties.

Sex toys, unlike many other aspects of sex, can be purely physical.

Sex toys can literally give you the sensation that no human can do for you or for her, and there's nothing wrong with that.

Nipple clamps, whips for spanking, blindfolds, and ties all do things for us that would be physically impossible otherwise – and in this way, it allows us to explore our sexuality and boundaries to how we might be fully satisfied.

But of course, there are psychological elements as well.

When you use these toys on a woman, it is all about getting her to visualize and live in that very special sexual environment that you are creating together. You want to be in this environment that has elements of danger, unconventionality, doing things that you aren't supposed to be doing, emotional urgency, and intimacy.

You have to remember that people who are into domination, or having their wife beat them or whip them around in bed, do so because they have a high level of trust. You trust your partner to not cross the line between exciting you and getting you off sexually, and outright physically abusing you.

That danger involved with trust is what makes kinky sex so appealing to so many Americans. It is really an exercise in trust. The fact that your partner wouldn't violate that trust makes you emotionally closer to her or, if you are a female, him.

You have to understand the emotional and psychological meanings of these toys. Vibrators, dildos, beads, clamps, whips, blindfolds, ties: they don't exist in a vacuum. They are not emotionally neutral.

Successfully integrating sex toys with sex.

The biggest mistake people have with sex toys is that they think sex toys replace sex. Instead of looking at them as props, they look at them as the complete production in themselves. This is like watching Les Mis and mistaking the background props for the actors.

Well, that is what you are doing if you are simply pleasing your partner with a sex toy. That defeats the whole purpose. The whole purpose is not the vibrator getting her off. That is not the whole purpose. The purpose is to integrate the vibrator with sex with you.

You have to agree with your partner as to how these toys would integrate with sex. And, the end result must be pleasurable to both of you on all levels. I am talking about a physically gratifying experience, an emotionally fulfilling experience, and a psychologically meaningful experience.

Otherwise, you are just wasting your time. Otherwise, you are falling into the very common mistake of using the sex toy as a sexual replacement. This can endanger your relationship. You can't help but feel emotionally torn up when you notice that your woman is pleasuring herself with a vibrator without you, and INSTEAD of you.

The whole point of the vibrator is to stimulate her while you are there, while she is in the process of having sex with you.

Fortunately, this is very simple to do. Just hold the vibrator on her clitoris while you fuck her, or tell her to hold it on herself. This will take her pleasure to the next level.

Sex toys for men: cock rings.

Cock rings are just what they sound like – it is commonly a ring of rubber that you put over your cock (and balls). This has a few beneficial effects when it comes to sex.

First, it makes you harder. The reason rubber works well as a cock ring is because it traps blood in your penis, and keeps you erect. It doesn't let blood leave it, yet it still allows blood to enter it and make your cock more engorged. This means that you are bigger during sex, and can do sex positions that you might not be able to when you aren't as hard.

Second, it can help with premature ejaculation. It literally is a barrier that clamps on your urethra at the base of your penis, so you can imagine how this can keep you from ejaculating when you don't want to.

Third, it makes you more sensitive during sex, on account of there being more blood in your penis. Obviously this makes sex a more pleasurable experience as a whole.

A variation on the cock ring is that some of them vibrate. This will vary from man to man if you enjoy the sensation of a vibrator on your cock, but know that it will definitely increase the pleasure for your woman. Every thrust she will essentially get her clitoris vibrated on – something to consider.

## 16. Multiple orgasms, you, and her.

You have probably come across some girls who say that they have a tough time orgasming. You probably have met or heard of at least one woman who has never ejaculated in her life. This really is too bad, because these women don't understand that they are blessed sexually.

If they come across a partner who knows what he is doing, or they open themselves up psychologically and emotionally to the fullest dimensions of sex, they can experience multiple orgasms. This is a unique and distinct blessing for women because, for the most part, men are not built that way.

We are not multi-load shotguns where you shoot off a load, then you cock it a little bit, you stick it back in, then you shoot off another load. We don't have the equipment for that. Women do, especially when it comes to clitoral stimulation.

In fact, one of the pieces of advice I give in this book is that you can actually make a woman come many times over - we are talking up to a dozen times in one night - by simply switching between clitoral, vaginal, and G-spot stimulation. If you have put in the right amount of time and effort into exploring your woman's G-spot, you are in luck.

Once you get her to come by stimulating the G-spot, you can switch back to stimulating her clit and have her come that way. Once she orgasms, then you switch back to the G-spot. You can keep doing this over and over until she passes out with a big smile on her face.

Multiple orgasms are a blessing. For men, on the other hand, you don't have this privilege. But, thanks to Kegel exercises and tantra, you can maximize your orgasm. The good news for guys is that, even though we only have one shot, we can make it an earth-shattering shot, as long as we go through the right exercises and have the right mind frame.

Keep the following considerations in mind, when it comes to multiple orgasms for both you and your partner.

Maximize your kegel strength to keep from coming quickly.

The biggest challenge to guys is not ejaculation. Guys are so horny that they can ejaculate at the drop of a hat.

Just flash the right porno and you can see guys rush to the bathroom to get themselves off.

The problem is: coming too quickly. Unfortunately, guys have low expectations when it comes to orgasms. They think that, as long as that fluid comes out of their penises and they get this rush from the base of their spines to the bottom part of their brains, they are good to go.

If that is your definition of a great orgasm, you are missing out.

Work out your kegels every day. Do sets of 20 throughout the day, and once you are comfortable with that, start holding and squeezing for two seconds for each repetition.

The big payoff here is that the longer you stay hard and keep yourself from coming, the better it is for your female partner. What is the payoff to you?

The big payoff to you is that your ejaculation, when it does come, is more intense. It is more fulfilling and it lasts longer. If you have a strong muscle that delivers your ejaculate, the feeling will be correspondingly strong.

Guys who work on ejaculating as quickly as possible have a very short enjoyment period for their climax. They come and ejaculate, and it lasts, at most, a few minutes. Wouldn't it be amazing to make that last ten, twenty minutes, or even an hour?

The good news is that through kegel exercises, you can

prolong the stimulation of your penis so that when you do ejaculate, it would be a very intense and memorable experience. Imagine you are having sex, and you are reaching the point of no return. Fortunately, you have worked on your kegels for weeks, and they are now rock solid. So when the feeling of orgasm comes, you can literally hold the ejaculate inside you because your kegels are so strong.

This keeps you hard, yet it still gives you the pleasure of an orgasm.

Not bad.

## 17. Dos and don'ts post-sex.

Now that you've had sex with your partner, it would be tempting to call it a night, roll over and go to sleep. If that is your attitude, then you are just like a typical guy and, guess what, most women complain about this typical guy behavior. What you do after sex is just as important as what you do before and during sex.

If you want to get invited back to the party, if you want to have sex with that amazing person again and again in the future, you have to pay serious attention to what you do after sex.

You have to remember that the female mind, as I mentioned in Chapter 1, is all about security, comfort, and trust. She wants to feel appreciated. She wants to feel that she belongs. She wants to feel protected.

This is very important to know, going into sex, doing sex, and emerging out of sex. If you don't conduct yourself in such a way, after sex, with these values in mind, then sex would essentially be meaningless to her.

It gives her the wrong kind of signals and decreases the likelihood that you would have sex with her again.

Do stay awake.

It is very common for guys to experience orgasm and feel tapped out.

If you had a particularly strong orgasm - we are talking about orgasm you achieve thanks to kegel exercises - you will feel really drained. It is very easy for you to have a long night's restful sleep after great sex.

However, you should resist rolling over and falling asleep. Instead, you need to stay awake and you need to devote the next hour, at least, to her needs. Only after she has fallen asleep would it be OK for you to fall asleep.

Remember, for guys, the secret to great sex is to reframe sex as an exercise not about your needs, but about hers. This is the best way for you to get invited back to the party, and to have sex with her again and again and again in the future.

Do cuddle.

Many guys are afraid of this. The reason they are afraid is that they are looking at sex as primarily something they physically do with a woman. Once they do it, they are out. I am sorry to break this to you, but you cannot do things that way. You have to make her feel appreciated, respected, loved and protected.

The best way to this is to simply spoon with her. With her turned to the side, you turn your front to her, wrap your legs around her, and hug her from the back. Wrap your face in her hair. Smell the back of her neck. Kiss her gently. Make her feel warm. Make her feel loved. Wrap her with your essence and your protection.

Just give her a little space if she needs for the sweat to dry.

<u>Don't fall asleep.</u>

When you fall asleep after sex, you are showing disrespect. You are showing her, in no uncertain terms, that her pleasure doesn't matter as much as yours. You are showing her that your needs come first before hers.

Notice my wording? Notice that I say the word "show" a lot? There is a reason for this. Women aren't dumb animals. You can say "I love you" all you want. You can say "I treasure and care, and cherish you" all you want. But your real motivations and your real intent speak loudly through your actions.

By falling asleep, you are basically slapping your partner in the face and telling her in a loud voice, "I used you and now I am done with you." That is precisely the wrong message you want to send. At the very least, she won't want to have sex with you again. At the very worst, you are doing yourself a big disservice, because you might be cutting off what would otherwise be great relationships, because of this bad habit.

## Don't lie still.

Right after sex, you may be awake. But if you just keep to yourself, or lie still flat on your back without touching your partner, that is just as bad as falling asleep.

Your partner is in a very sensitive state right after sex. She is highly excited on many different levels. Emotionally, she is engaged. Psychologically, she is opened up. Spiritually, she is in tune. Physically, she is raw and sensitive.

She needs your warm touch. She needs your presence. She needs you to be there. By lying still on your back, you are basically telling her to forget you. "I got what I want from you. Now leave me alone." That is not a good move.

## Do clean her off.

Sex isn't a super clean act. Of course, most of the time when we're in the moment we don't notice, or don't care about this at all. We're pursuing a greater goal at the time, and who cares about a little bit of bodily fluid?

But the second after we orgasm and finish, our mindset changes drastically. Suddenly, we're sticky and wet all over!

Your girl will also feel this way, and she knows she will have to clean herself up all over after the deed.

So after sex, take the initiative to help clean her off! Give her a wet paper towel or towel, wipe her off, walk her through the nuances of your bathroom, turn the fan on, and whatever else to make her feel comfortable and taken care of after the fact.

Remember guys, it's psychological, so when she sees you taking care of her in such basic ways, she will appreciate it so much and feel strongly towards you as a man.

## Conclusion

Now that we've learned all about the basics of sex, and how to skyrocket your woman's pleasure and make her scream... it's just a matter of putting it into practice!

I wish you the best, and I know that your woman will feel her best from this day forward.

Make me proud and make her scream.

Love,

Amber Cole

Printed in Great Britain
by Amazon